4324

THE POISON CONSPIRACY

Also by Karl Grossman

COVER UP: What you *are not* supposed to know
about Nuclear Power

The Poison Conspiracy

Karl Grossman

Illustrations by
Van Howell

THE PERMANENT PRESS
Sag Harbor, N.Y. 11963

Edited by Janet Grossman

International Standard Book Number: 0-932966-26-8
Library of Congress Catalog Card Number: 82-083124
The Permanent Press, Sag Harbor, New York 11963
Printed in the United States of America

For Janet

"The earth is mine sayeth the Lord, and ye are but stewards."

Leviticus

Contents

Introduction

The merchandising of poison has become a huge global growth industry.

> **POISON:** Any agent which introduced into an organism may chemically produce an injurious or deadly effect.
>
> Webster's Dictionary

Many toxins are peddled to specifically kill, but poison is hardly ever *specific* so these poisons—pesticides to kill insects, herbicides to kill plants, for example—spread injury and death far beyond their targets. In addition, there are the poisons sold for another purpose—such as additives to preserve, treat or color food. In sufficient quantities these additives produce injury and death. And there are the poisons generated as by-products of industrial processes which pollute the air, the water, the earth and also reap their deadly harvest.

That the world is being poisoned, that as a principal result cancer is spreading in epidemic proportions, and that life is being lost on a wide scale, is something more and more people have become aware of—often painfully.

What we have not become sufficiently aware of is that virtually nothing is being done to stop the poisoning. This is because the distribution of poison has become a powerful institution and a business. Protection by government is a sham.

1

That is what this book is primarily about: the Poison Conspiracy. It is about the government agencies which are supposed to protect us from poisons but do not because of the power of the industries involved in producing chemical poisons. These corporations have been able to warp, distort and neutralize those social mechanisms of protection—from local health departments to national enforcement bodies—which are supposed to function along the lines of that ancient human survival drive: the avoidance of poison.

It is about why the *Silent Spring* that Rachel Carson wrote about two decades ago *is still with us,* indeed *increasingly* with us, and how our health and lives are not being guarded.

As this federal government report, *Cancer-Causing Chemicals In Food,* declared:

DEAR CHAIRMAN STAGGERS: The attached report by the Subcommittee on Oversight and Investigations reviews the Federal government's efforts to protect the public from potentially dangerous amounts of pesticide residues in food. It focuses on the activities of the Environmental Protection Agency (EPA), Department of Agriculture (USDA), and the Food and Drug Administration (FDA) with regard to pesticide tolerance setting, residue monitoring, and enforcement of statutes designed to keep unhealthy levels of pesticides from being deposited on or in food products.

The Subcommittee concludes that these programs are inadequate. As a result, American consumers cannot be sure that the meat, poultry, fruits, and vegetables they buy are not tainted with potentially dangerous pesticide residues.

We all have to eat. Because of the nature of chemical contaminants, we are forced to rely on the Federal government to protect us against potentially dangerous chemicals we cannot see, smell, or taste. Our examination leads us to believe that we cannot rely on the Federal government to protect us.

We found for instance that EPA (1) continues to approve tolerances for potentially carcinogenic, mutagenic, and teratogenic pesticides which result in residues in or on food; (2) has set tolerances for some of these pesticides without complete safety data; (3) has exempted some potentially dangerous pesticides from its tolerance requirements which end up in or on food; (4) uses an inadequate and outdated statistical base for setting tolerance levels; (5) often does not know what level of pesticide residue usually results from the use of a product; and (6) bases its approval of pesticides merely on industry-supplied safety data which often does not fully examine the potential hazard posed by the pesticide.

CANCER-CAUSING CHEMICALS IN FOOD

REPORT

together with

SEPARATE VIEWS

BY THE

SUBCOMMITTEE ON OVERSIGHT AND INVESTIGATIONS

OF THE

COMMITTEE ON INTERSTATE AND FOREIGN COMMERCE

NINETY-FIFTH CONGRESS

SECOND SESSION

DECEMBER 1978

. . . American consumers cannot be sure that the meat, poultry, fruits, and vegetables they buy are not tainted with potentially dangerous pesticide residues.

We all have to eat. Because of the nature of chemical contaminants, we are forced to rely on the Federal government to protect us against potentially dangerous chemicals we cannot see, smell, or taste. Our examination leads us to believe that we cannot rely on the Federal government to protect us.

And notice, the EPA *continues to approve tolerances for potentially carcinogenic, mutagenic, and teratogenic pesticides which result in residues in or on food. It has set tolerances for some of these pesticides without complete safety data, has exempted some potentially dangerous pesticides from its tolerance requirements which end up in or on food, uses an inadequate and outdated statistical base for setting tolerance levels, often does not know what level of pesticide residue usually results from the use of a product. Moreover it bases its approval of pesticides merely on industry-supplied safety data which often does not fully examine the potential hazard posed by the pesticide.*
And—

In sum, the Subcommittee concludes that EPA's tolerance setting program is abysmal and needs a complete overhaul.

Additionally, the Subcommittee is alarmed with the inadequate monitoring and enforcement programs of USDA and FDA. The Subcommittee found that even when meat was found to be contaminated with dangerously high levels of toxic pesticides neither USDA nor FDA could stop these products from reaching the dinner table. This is an appalling state of affairs which cannot be allowed to continue.

The investigatory panel declared:

Chapter V—General Conclusion

The Subcommittee on Oversight and Investigations concludes that the federal programs designed to protect the American public from toxic chemicals in food, which are administered jointly by the United States Department of Agriculture (USDA), the Environmental Protection Agency (EPA), and the Food and Drug Administration (FDA), are ineffective. In some cases, existing laws need amending. (Recommendations for new legislation are presented at the close of the three chapters on agency programs.) However, in many more instances, the EPA, FDA and USDA are failing to carry out the vital responsibilities invested in them to protect the public from dangerous chemical residues in food. These failures are briefly summarized here:

EPA: The federal chemical residue monitoring system hinges on a strong pesticide tolerance setting program. However, the Environmental Protection Agency's system for setting tolerances (safe, legal limits of chemical residues that may be found in specific foods) is outdated, ineffectual, and showing few signs of improvement, EPA's Office of Pesticide Programs is veering away from the health-oriented language of the Federal Food, Drug, and Cosmetic Act, which administers the tolerance setting program, toward the "risk-benefit" balancing language of the Federal Insecticide, Fungicide and Rodenticide Act, under which pesticides are registered for use. In so doing, the EPA is putting the public at greater risk. Many tolerances remain in effect for pesticides that are known to be suspect carcinogens. Scores of other tolerances are for chemicals that have never been tested for carcinogenicity or other equally serious effects.

USDA: The United States Department of Agriculture, which is responsible for monitoring meat and poultry for residues of chemicals such as pesticides and animal drugs, is doing a poor job of finding residue violations and of preventing (in conjunction with the Food and Drug Administration) the marketing of contaminated meat. The Department's two residue monitoring programs (on the farm and in the slaughterhouse) are seriously ineffective. The "in slaughterhouse" monitoring program tests few animals and doesn't look for many harmful chemicals known to occur in meat and poultry. The "pretest" program, which enjoins growers suspected of marketing violative livestock to submit tissue samples for laboratory analysis, is easily avoided by farmers. Consequently, much of the meat and poultry consumed in this country may be contaminated. The USDA inspection stamp goes on all produce that has passed inspection for *visible* signs of health and cleanliness. The stamp is no guarantee that meat is free of chemical contaminants.

FDA: The Food and Drug Administration's role in the regulation of toxic substances in food includes monitoring agricultural produce (other than meat and poultry) for residues of pesticides and environmental contaminants, investigating and prosecuting cases of residue violations in meat and poultry reported to FDA by USDA, and sharing responsibility, with USDA, for keeping contaminated produce out of interstate commerce. FDA's chemical monitoring program has dangerous shortcomings. Many chemicals occurring in food that are known to be suspect carcinogens or may potentially cause birth defects and genetic mutations are not monitored. FDA investigates few of the residue violations reported to it by USDA and rarely prosecutes violators. Combined USDA-FDA programs to remove contaminated meat from the marketplace almost never result in meat or poultry recalls.

And all this was before Ronald Reagan began systematically dismantling what regulatory function there was in federal government.

Consider this report:

BY THE COMPTROLLER GENERAL

Report To The Congress

OF THE UNITED STATES

EPA Is Slow To Carry Out Its Responsibility To Control Harmful Chemicals

For almost 4 years EPA has had broad authority to protect the public and the environment from the harmful effects of chemicals. Although actions have been taken to control three chemicals, no chemicals have been tested and basic data is lacking on most of the other 55,000 chemicals now in use. New chemicals are being screened, but implementing regulations and the review process itself have not been completed.

Several factors have contributed to this slow progress, including no clear sense of direction to guide the program, and organizational and staffing problems. EPA is working to resolve these problems.

CED-81-1
OCTOBER 28, 1980

What a track record! *Although actions have been taken to control three chemicals, no chemicals have been tested and basic data is lacking on most of the other 55,000 chemicals now in use.*

As this report summarized:

D I G E S T

The Toxic Substances Control Act of 1976 gave the Environmental Protection Agency (EPA) a broad mandate to protect the public and the environment from unreasonable chemical risks. However, almost 4 years later, neither the public nor the environment are much better protected.

Or consider this report:

BY THE COMPTROLLER GENERAL

Report To The Congress
OF THE UNITED STATES

Stronger Enforcement Needed Against Misuse Of Pesticides

Programs enforcing Federal pesticide laws are key factors in making sure that the public and the environment are not unnecessarily exposed to hazardous pesticides. But these programs have not always been adequate. For example, the Environmental Protection Agency and the States do not always properly investigate cases and sometimes take questionable enforcement actions.

EPA and States also have problems with the special registration program. In some cases, State agencies may be circumventing pesticide laws.

EPA and States need to alleviate the problems that continue to plague the enforcement programs and improve their management to help ensure the public's protection.

CED-82-5
OCTOBER 15, 1981

Here the Comptroller General declares that its General Accounting Office found that the

public may not always be protected from pesticide misuse because EPA and the States

--sometimes take questionable enforcement actions against violators,

--have not implemented adequate program administration and monitoring, and

--are approving the use of pesticides for special local needs and emergency purposes which may be circumventing EPA's normal pesticide registration procedures.

LACK OF ADEQUATE
ENFORCEMENT ACTIONS

EPA and State enforcement programs do not always protect the public and the environment because:

--Many enforcement actions are questionable or inconsistent. (See p. 9.)

--Some cases are poorly investigated. (See p. 12.)

--State lead agencies often do not share EPA's enforcement philosophy. (See p. 14.)

--Most States lack the ability to impose civil penalties. (See p. 15.)

Under the Reagan administration, things have gotten worse—although they were horrendous before.

Now the Poison Conspiracy has become thoroughly obvious.

Examine the top ranks of a principal would-be protective agency, the EPA.

"The chemical industry has been given an important role in the Reagan Administration's selection of a new chief of the EPA," reported the *Washington Post* in January 1981. Chosen EPA administrator was Anne Gorsuch, a telephone company lawyer and state legislator from Colorado who consistently supported polluting industry and was pivotal in killing a state program to deal with toxic wastes.

"FOXES IN CHARGE OF EPA'S EGGS," headlined the *Atlantic Constitution* in July 1981 noting that of those people Mrs. Gorsuch decided to surround herself with "eleven of the first fifteen subordinates named are former lawyers, lobbyists or consultants from industries which the EPA regulates. Included are representatives from major industries that often have pollution problems, like steel, oil, coal, paper and chemicals. In several instances former industry representatives run programs that they sought to make less stringent before they joined the EPA."

"These are people who have worked for industries that are opposed to what EPA is trying to do," said William Butler of the National Audubon Society. "The regulated have captured the regulators."

● Robert M. Perry, a veteran lawyer for the Exxon oil company in Houston, was named EPA general counsel.

● Dr. John Todhunter, a long-time representative of opponents of restrictions on pesticides and "scientific advisor" of the industry-financed American Council on Science and Health, was picked as assistant administrator for pesticides and toxic substances.

● Kathleen Bennett who, as her official EPA biography reads, "for many years prior to joining EPA served as Washington representative"—a lobbyist—"for industries having strong environmental concerns and impact," including the American Paper Institute and Crown Zellerbach as they fought to weaken the Clean Air Act, was named assistant administrator for air pollution control programs, to supervise the Clean Air Act.

• John E. Daniel, who as a lawyer in Washington represented the Manville Corporation and defended its products, including cancer-causing asbestos, before the EPA and other government agencies in Washington and before that was also a Washington lobbyist—"director of environmental and legislative affairs"—for the American Paper Institute, was picked as Mrs. Gorsuch's chief of staff.

• Rita Lavelle, a public relations person for the Aerojet-General Corporation, a chemical/aerospace conglomerate involved in hazardous waste-dumping and pollution of water in California, was named assistant administrator for solid waste and emergency response, to direct the "Superfund" hazardous waste program.

• Nolan E. Clark whose Washington law firm represented Dow Chemical before the EPA and other agencies in Dow's battle against any restrictions on commercial use of the herbicide 2,4,5-T—a basic ingredient of Agent Orange—was appointed associate administrator for policy and resource management.

• Frank Shepherd, a lawyer who represented General Motors, a leading opponent of the Clean Air Act, was named associate administrator for legal counsel and enforcement.

• William Sullivan, Jr., a lawyer who ran a consulting firm involving the steel industry which fought against environmental controls for steel mills, was named deputy associate administrator for legal counsel and enforcement.

"If I were an environmental activist, I'd be scared to death," Sullivan said of his appointment.

"These people owe their allegience not to the American public but to their former corporate employers and benefactors," says John P. Shea, former counsel to the Council on Environmental Quality.

And who did President Reagan appoint as chairman of the President's Cancer Panel? None other than Armand Hammer, chairman of Occidental Petroleum which owns Hooker Chemicals and Plastics Company—the corporation which gave us Love Canal and other toxic waste disasters that have resulted in a high incidence of cancer among local residents.

But, as Hugh B. Kaufman, an EPA toxic waste expert and one of the few people of integrity in government trying to do

something about the poisoning which has been allowed to
become pervasive, says: "I'm not sure that government at any
level has the wherewithall to stand up to the large generator
companies, the generators of toxic waste. And that's really
where the rub comes in.

"When you have the largest companies in the world pres-
suring the federal government," he continues, a situation results which "pretty much wouldn't change from administration to administration."

The Reagan administrators are "more venal and so their
tactics for imposing their will tend to be a little blunter" than
the Carter administrators, for example, but "the end-result is
probably the same," Kaufman concludes.

Declares another EPA whistle-blower, William Sanjour:
"Depending on the federal government to regulate things is
absolutely worthless. They just make matters worse." As to
the Carter and Reagan administrations, "they are about the
same," he says.

In fact, instead of emphasizing that poisoning stop, the
would-be protective measures by government have been
translated into regulation has, which has, in effect, led to the
licensing of poisoning.

"It gives license to continue to pollute and actually makes it
easier to continue to pollute by doing it under federal auspices," says Sanjour, chief of the EPA's hazardous waste
implementation branch.

Lorna Salzman of Friends of the Earth points out: "The real
question is who, and by what authority, can have the power to
determine how many illnesses and deaths are acceptable? "If
someone conspired to kill another, then that person would be
"legally culpable," she notes. But "corporations involved in
the manufacture and use of poison on the general populace
can do this under the umbrella of regulation. The fact that the
names of the victims are not known makes it legal but I don't
think there's a distinction. Those deaths are statistically certain and morally there is no difference. Society cannot permit
random, premeditated murder. It cannot delegate the moral
and ethical power to decide life and death in the name of
private profit."

The creation of government regulatory agencies has been

the "best thing" for corporations, she says, because these agencies "legitamatize and rationalize" the illnesses and death caused by these companies.

There is no need to "set standards for and regulate" the output of poison, says Mrs. Salzman. Poison simply should be subject to an "outright ban" and those people, those "heads of companies" whose activities and toxins result in illness and death should be subject to criminal sanctions—"like all individuals who assault and kill."

To know what we face is important. To know what has to be done and what is not being done, to know about the puffery and *the charade that passes for protection,* is just as important.

And to know there are abundant *alternatives* to dirtying our nest, spreading toxins, poisoning the planet—that none of this is necessary other than for the profit and power of those institutions and people that do it—this, too, is vital for our survival.

These are all the reasons this book is written.

KARL GROSSMAN

Sag Harbor, New York
January, 1983

On Poison's Front Line

Among the people most heavily-hit by cancer and other so-called environmental diseases—maladies caused by poisons put into the environment—are those who live near toxic waste dumps, people who live near factories where toxins are spewed out into the air, land and water, workers in industries where poisons are prevalent, and farmers and farmworkers heavily involved with chemical pesticides, herbicides and fertilizers.

***

"I have very bad feelings about the government now and I just didn't before," Anne Anderson of Woburn, Massachusetts is saying. The Anderson family lives a little more than a mile from a waste dump. In 1972, Billy Anderson, then but three and a half, was diagnosed as having leukemia. In January 1981 he died—ravaged by the disease, just four feet three inches tall at twelve and a half, and weighing fifty-two pounds; he had lost his hair three separate times.

Since 1969 eight children who live in homes near the Woburn dump have died from leukemia. "Another one was diagnosed a couple of months ago," says Mrs. Anderson in 1982. "It still seems to be going on."

Woburn, 12 miles north of Boston, has the highest death rate from cancer of any community in Massachusetts. Besides the leukemia deaths, over twice the national average, the kidney cancer level is nearly twice the U.S. rate. The incidence of cancer of the liver, bronchus, lung, breast, prostate, pancreas and stomach are also abnormally high in this town of 35,000.

"I went through an awful lot of suffering. I saw my son suffer an awful lot for nine years, I mean it was constant," says Mrs. Anderson. And with just a few exceptions (notably Senator Edward Kennedy, she says) "there just wasn't anybody that wanted to listen."

The dump has been in Woburn since 1853 and was used at one time by the leading U.S. producer of ingredients for arsenic-based pesticides. Tanneries, a glue-making factory, and other chemical companies have discharged their poisons into the dump. Its 60 acres of hills, lakes and fields are thoroughly contaminated with toxics including arsenic, lead and chromium. In 1979, it was discovered that water in wells near the dump supplying Mrs. Anderson's neighborhood were extensively poisoned with such carcinogenic substances as trichloroethylene and chloroform.

Mrs. Anderson says that after it was found that her son had leukemia, the family considered a link with the "foul-tasting, foul-smelling, foul-looking water we had been subjected to," and when "a neighbor came and said two other children in the neighborhood" also had leukemia, the Andersons suspected the leukemia was connected to the dump and the bad water.

But "we couldn't get anybody willing to admit that the water was an influence in the sickness," recounts Mrs. Anderson.

Mrs. Anderson says "initially I didn't know where to go. You just turn to your local board of health, your local politicians and they just keep telling us that the water was potable, that there was no problem with the water."

Later, the Massachusetts Department of Environmental Quality was persuaded to get involved, and it said it would do studies. In 1982, "they're about to start testing" at the dump, says Mrs. Anderson. "It's been taking years."

The week Jimmy died, Massachusetts Health Commissioner Alfred Frechette issued a report declaring that there were "no positive leads or associations" connecting toxic waste contamination in Woburn and its spiraling cancer rate.

EPA has been "cooperative to a certain point, but only to a

point, I think, to appease us," Mrs. Anderson continues. "I can't see that they're really being aggressive about finding a link or a cause or any tie-in with health problems at all. And they'll say that that's really not their area."

Does she think, after her experiences, that government agencies protect people?

"No, I don't," she says. "It's up to the citizen, at his own expense, on his own time, to try to prove that there is a health hazard, that there are chemicals that could be injurious to health and instead of really having someone that the public can go to and expect to listen, they don't listen. They don't want to hear it. They don't want to know there's a problem. This is on the local and state and federal level. They just don't want to hear it."

Why does she believe this is so?

"I think they see dollars, and I think they see industry being hurt and that, of course, is uppermost in the minds of our government. Everything hinges on how well business is doing. But I think if they really inquire about the health effects that people are suffering and the money that that's ultimately costing the government, they'd find they're really not looking close enough at the dollar signs."

Sometimes agency representatives who cover the area will conduct meetings. "They'll sit down, every once in a while, and they'll talk to you. But they're talking for the government and they're really talking in circles. They're not receptive to things. They'll tell you, 'Well, if you think something, come and tell us.' And you tell them and nothing gets done anyway. I'm really to the point where I said to one of them last week, 'Do we have to scream and bang on doors?' I mean, we've taken the tack for so many years of being really cooperative and quietly doing what we can and really not getting in their way, but it's been just years and so little has been done. All that's been done in the industrial park is a fence. They put a fence around it after several years—several years," repeats Mrs. Anderson, who has co-founded a group called FACE (For A Cleaner Environment). It had just begun a house-by-house illness survey of Woburn.

"We lost three children last year, another one is in critical condition now," she continues. The string of leukemia deaths near the Woburn dump "can't be just chalked up to a fluke."

Mrs. Anderson, pain in her voice, declares: "You see it with the Agent Orange. How much does government do for the men who suffer the effects of Agent Orange, or for that matter radiation? It just doesn't make any sense. I don't understand. I always thought this country, this government was humane. I was a child of the Second World War, and my first memories were of the good guys, the Americans. And I just always felt that we had a humane government and that they were looking out for us, be it at the cookie factory level or whatever. And to find out they turn their backs on the people who are suffering!

"I've had to do a complete about-face," she says, her voice breaking, "to the point where I don't want my other son to . . . I don't think he should . . .fight for this government. Ask me ten years ago and I, of course, I didn't feel this way. I have very negative feelings towards the government because I don't think it needed to be and I think if they are on top of things, it wouldn't happen."

***

"I'm worried and very angry," Karen Levinson is saying. "I feel that the agencies that are there to protect us are not doing the job they're supposed to be doing."

Mrs. Levinson lives a block and a half from a plant in Hicksville, New York long used by the Hooker Chemicals and Plastics Company to make a vinyl chloride resin used as a "plasticizer" in the manufacture of plastic-coated drinking cups and elastic for panty hose.

Like so much of the rest of Hooker's operations—from Love Canal, New York to Montague, Michigan to Bloody Run Creek, New York to White Lake, Michigan to Taft, Louisiana to Jacksonville, Florida—Hooker's Hicksville operation has been filthy.

Reported a 1980 study entitled *Toxics On Tap,* done by the Toxic Chemicals Project of the New York Public Interest Research Group (NYPIRG):

Hooker Chemicals and Plastics-RUCO Division
SPDES permit number: NY 0104388
New South Road
Hicksville, NY 11802

This facility is the largest known source of toxic organic chemical groundwater contamination on Long Island. For a detailed discussion of its polyester, plasticizer and urethane manufacturing operations and a description of the wide variety of highly toxic wastes that have been generated and disposed of improperly in recent decades, refer to this plant's profile in the hazardous waste landfill section of this report.

At present all liquid process wastes are fed into concrete holding tanks and then into an incinerator at a rate of 4,000 gallons per day. The incinerator burns the wastes at a temperature of approximately 1400°F. An assessment of the incinerator's potential as a source of air-borne toxic chemical pollution needs to be undertaken. It is possible that a portion of toxic organic wastes subjected to thermal destruction in the incinerator are not exposed to temperatures capable of causing total molecular breakdown. These compounds could volatilize and escape into the atmosphere.

The report was highly critical of the permit New York State granted Hooker to allow it to discharge poisons at its Hicksville operation under the State Pollutant Discharge Elimination System, or SPEDES.
It stressed:

The Hooker plant site is contaminated with tons of some of the most toxic chemicals known to exist. Many of the toxics are capable of migrating throughout the groundwater system, causing widespread contamination. Thus far, however, a full assessment of the site's pollution potential has not been undertaken. Nor have sophisticated monitoring systems been employed to determine precisely where the pollution has reached. Consequently, though the site may be assumed to be extremely contaminated, there is no accurate way to calculate precisely how seriously this site threatens the public health of the area's residents.

Mrs. Levinson, at 28, developed cervical cancer in 1980. She underwent a hysterectomy and now lives in constant fear for the health of her entire family. "I'm afraid what will happen to my children, the possible effects it will have.

"Hooker Chemical spews smoke out in the air on a nightly basis," she says. Sometimes it is "a fog of smoke you can't see through." And the company, she says, has stubbornly refused to disclose what exactly it has been discharging.

As to government protection, "I feel we're being ignored," says Mrs. Levinson. Government—from the federal to the local level—seems to not care about what Hooker has been up to.

"The bottom line," says Walter Hang, staff scientist on the *Toxics On Tap* study, "is that industries in America have been able to get their way and environmental programs have not made the kind of progress that we once thought that they would be able to make ten years ago when they were instituted. As a result, the environment gets more contaminated on a day-to-day basis.

"Even today, if I wanted to start up a chemical corporation in America and wanted to discharge hundreds of millions of gallons of contaminated wastewater loaded with the deadliest poisons known to exist, I could get a permit from the EPA or from a state authority and that permit would not restrict me from discharging PCB's, dioxin, arguably the deadliest chemical know to man, and so on.

"The corporations," says Hang, "will basically say anything to benefit themselves and to maximize their profits. They don't want to stop dumping the toxic chemicals; they don't want to be held liable for the types of problems they have created."

"It's a situation," Hang continues, that "goes all the way from the top down. At the highest levels of government you have politicians who many times are put in office through large contributions of major corporations" and these same corporations, often through trade associations, have been easily able to block efforts by regulatory agencies.

Toxics On Tap declared:

Americans take clean drinking water for granted. When a twist of the faucet brings it pouring out, there is no visible indication that it is scarce or unhealthy. Knowing very little about where their drinking water comes from or how it is purified, most people assume it is abundant and, for the most part, safe to drink. This opinion is widely held despite unmistakable signs that water quality is not what it used to be. In recent years all too many of the nation's rivers and lakes have been discovered to be highly contaminated with toxic chemicals. Vast bodies of water, including the Hudson River and Lake Ontario, are now known to be thoroughly polluted with millions of tons of raw industrial wastes. Fish and wildlife living in these waters accumulate the poisonous substances in their flesh and are inedible. Most importantly, drinking water drawn from these sources is also tainted. Since the techniques used to purify water in this country essentially date from the 19th century, when man-made chemicals did not exist, they are incapable of removing water-borne synthetic organic compounds. Consequently these pollutants are consumed in drinking water by millions of people every day. The public health implications of this problem are undeniably frightening.

Nationwide, over 700 chemical pollutants have been identified in public water supplies. Most of these are cancer-causing (carcinogenic), cause birth defects (teratogenic) or are otherwise toxic. Over 20 scientific studies have documented a consistent link between consumption of trace organic chemical contaminants in drinking water and elevated cancer mortality rates. In spite of mounting evidence, existing United States public health standards reflect virtually no concern for toxic and carcinogenic substances in drinking water. As a result no concerted effort has been made to remove them from public supplies. The parallel failures to protect drinking water quality and regulate massive discharges of non-biodegradable industrial wastes forecast a grim future. Invasive toxic contamination has already forced many communities to find alternative sources of water supply. Still, the overwhelming majority of the nation's drinking water systems have never been tested for the presence of toxic pollutants. Unquestionably, the response to this dual environmental/health dilemma has been woefully inadequate.

"Unless decisive action is taken soon," said *Toxics On Tap*, "America will pay dearly for its out-of-sight, out-of-mind approach to eliminating toxic chemical hazards."
Toxics On Tap emphasized:

> A myth is being perpetrated in this state that toxic chemical pollution is under control. In fact, little could be further from the truth. New York's agencies and the nation as a whole are in no way prepared for the on-coming environmental crisis. As this study shows, toxic chemical discharges from industries, dumps and developed areas are beyond the control of our existing health and environmental management programs. Unless fundamental reforms are implemented, the situation will only worsen in the years ahead as hundreds of tons of raw wastes are released into the air, land and water.

Out-of-control pollution is spreading cancer rampantly. From *Toxics On Tap:*

> Cancer is actually a group of over 100 illnesses resulting from the uncontrolled growth of cells. Normally the human body's billons of cells are specialized to accomplish exacting duties. The complex operation of organs and life processes are precisely regulated and harmonious with one another. When cancer develops, however, the effects are devastating. Cancerous cells disregard the body's internal system of operational controls. Growing at faster rates than normal, cancerous cells build up into tumors. These independent masses of cells invade, compress, and destroy surrounding tissues. Through the process of metastasis, cancerous cells spread throughout the bloodstream and lymph system to form new tumors elsewhere in the body. Ultimately, the body becomes so weakened that death occurs.
>
> Cancer ranks as the second leading cause of death in America. At its present rate cancer will afflict one out of every four citizens in the nation sometime during their lives. Approximately 54 million people alive at this time in the USA will someday get cancer. Two-thirds of those people will die from the disease. Only heart illness kills more people in America.
>
> The vastness of these statistics fails to convey the agony

and dread caused by cancer. Nevertheless, so many have died from this disease that the cancer experience of drawn-out pain and suffering is close to universal in our country. More people die annually from cancer than all the Americans who died in combat during the entire second World War. As a result there are few Americans who have not been touched in some way by cancer, their lives changed forever. The economic costs of cancer are also devastating. The direct and indirect costs of cancer have been calculated to range from $15 billion to $25 billion a year.

Environmental Cancer

The scientific community generally agrees that the majority of human cancers are environmentally induced. Estimates by the World Health Organization and the National Cancer Institute concur that between 60 and 90 percent of all human cancers are environmental in origin, and that approximately 90 percent of all human cancers are chemical in origin. These estimates have resulted from carefully conducted epidemiological investigations in the workplace, or in large diverse populations over the years.

Since the turn of the century, the incidence rate of cancer has risen steadily and drastically. In 1900 cancer was the eighth leading cause of death. Today it is number two. Between 1930 and 1975, the age-adjusted national cancer rate jumped from 116.7 deaths per 100,000 people to 130.9 deaths per 100,000. This increased toll is far above the rise expected from either the increased longevity of Americans, the decline of other leading causes of death (such as infectious diseases), the population boom or other related factors.

Ironically, cancer is a largely preventable hazard. Many sicknesses previously thought to arise spontaneously are now known to be caused by environmental pollution. This is especially true of cancer. Toxic substances, including carcinogens, are in the air we breathe, the food we eat, the consumer products we use and the water we drink. Exposure to these chemicals have significant deleterious effects on human health, most notably the incitement of tumors. Multiple exposures can exert additive, synergistic or antagonistic effects. Thus, as our environment grows increasingly contaminated with synthetic pollutants, the cancer risks we bear also rise.

This rise is a direct consequence of increased toxic chemical exposure. It is evident that cancer's general increase is closely parallel to the deterioration of the nation's environment. A graph of industrial activities known to be major contributors to toxic pollution follows a concurrent rising trend of cancer mortality. Loose in the environment, synthetic pollutants may not break down for decades. Instead they accumulate in "hot spots" or in the flesh of fish and wildlife. Human beings are similarly poisoned. Extremely carcinogenic or otherwise toxic compounds such as: polychlorinated biphenyls (PCB's), DDT, DDE, DDD, BHC (benzene hexachloride), aldrin/dieldrin, endrin, mirex, lindane, heptachlor, heptachlor epoxide, oxychlordane, hexachlorobenzene, transnonachlor, and dioxin have all been detected in American flesh.

It is highly probable, unfortunately, that so long as we increasingly expose ourselves to carcinogens in the environment, the rise in the cancer rate will continue correspondingly, for cancer is a latent disease. Once induced its symptoms may not appear for as long as 40 years. Presently observed cancer rates are generally the results of exposures that occurred decades ago. Logically, therefore, these rising trends can be extrapolated to much higher rates in the future.

Americans have yet to experience the full impact of heavy industry's massive expansion. Petrochemical production alone has skyrocketed by more than 2,000 per cent since the end of World War II. The country's production of synthetic organic chemicals has more than doubled in the last ten years. Over 334 million metric tons (wet) of industrial waste are generated annually in America, with a growth rate of 3 percent per year. The EPA estimates that up to 15 percent of that waste is hazardous and that more than 90 percent of the hazardous waste is dumped in unsafe ways each year. Consequently prospects for the future are grim. The worst health effects of industry's pollution of air, land and water will be felt in the coming decades.

A mammoth field of time-bombs has been planted, their full impacts yet to come, as *Toxics On Tap* stressed. *The worst health effects of industry's pollution of air, land and water will be felt in the coming decades*.

Hang had been a cancer researcher at Roswell Park Memorial Institute before joining NYPIRG as a staff scientist. "I decided to leave Roswell Park and stop trying to cure this disease which was essentially incurable and instead try to prevent the disease by making sure people are not exposed to toxic chemicals in their drinking water, work settings, by living in homes in heavily polluted areas," he says. By preventing pollution, people "will not get the cancers so we won't have to have them treated or cured, neither of which we can do anyway."

Hang says the solution to pollution is in democracy, of people saying, "I will not tolerate toxic chemicals in my drinking water."

He says: "What Americans have to get used to is the notion that corporations just can't be allowed to dump this stuff wherever they choose. When citizens begin to call for action, by the thousands, by the millions, that's when you'll be able to counter the political influence of multinational corporations which otherwise would dominate public policy."

"When you get enough people to say, 'We want to preserve the environment, we want to preserve our health by making sure we're not going to be exposed to toxic chemicals,' that's when," says Hang, "you begin to make the system work in your favor. I think that's possible." People must "band together and speak in one voice and say, 'We won't stand it anymore.'"

Mrs. Levinson has joined NYPIRG's campaign against toxic chemical pollution. "The only way people like myself can fight bureaucracy," she says, "is to get together."

***

Increasingly, workers in industries where poisons are common have been falling to cancer and other environmental disease.

"At least 20%" of the cancer in the U.S. is attributable to "occupational exposure," declared this 1978 report by the National Cancer Institute, National Institute of Environmental Health Sciences and National Institute for Occupational Safety and Health. And that, it said, may be a "conservative" figure.

ESTIMATES OF THE FRACTION OF
CANCER IN THE UNITED STATES
RELATED TO OCCUPATIONAL FACTORS

Prepared by:

National Cancer Institute
National Institute of Environmental Health Sciences
National Institute for Occupational Safety and Health

Contributors (alphabetical order):

Kenneth Bridbord, M.D., NIOSH
Pierre Decoufle, Sc.D., NCI
Joseph F. Fraumeni, Jr., M.D., NCI
David G. Hoel, Ph.D., NIEHS
Robert N. Hoover, M.D., Sc.D., NCI
David P. Rall, M.D., Ph.D., NIEHS, Director
Umberto Saffiotti, M.D., NCI
Marvin A. Schneiderman, Ph.D., NCI
Arthur C. Upton, M.D., NCI, Director

Contributor to the Appendix:

Nicholas Day, Ph.D., NCI, IARC

September 15, 1978

The report's summary included these points:

• Although exposure to some of the more important occupational carcinogens has been reduced in recent years, there are still many unregulated carcinogens in the U.S. workplaces; a number of occupations are characterized by excess cancer risks which have not yet been attributed to specific agents.

• There is no sound reason to assume that the future consequences of present-day exposure to carcinogens in the workplace will be less than those of exposure in the recent past.

• Patterns and trends in total cancer incidence (and mortality) in the U.S. are consistent with the hypothesis that occupationally-related cancers comprise a substantial and increasing fraction of total cancer incidence.

It concluded: "Occupationally-related cancers offer important opportunities for prevention."

A leading organization fighting occupationally-related cancers and other diseases has been the Oil, Chemical & Atomic Workers International Union.

Its monthly publication *LIFELINES* and its regular *ALERT* bulletins are constant and impeccably documented reports of the horror in much of the workplaces of America.

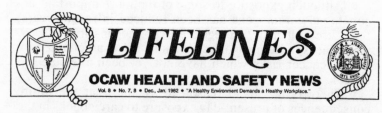

LIFELINES
OCAW HEALTH AND SAFETY NEWS
Vol. 8 • No. 7, 8 • Dec., Jan. 1982 • "A Healthy Environment Demands a Healthy Workplace."

Unions Join Forces on Formaldehyde
Petition OSHA for ETS

OCAW has joined the UAW and 11 other unions in petitioning OSHA for an Emergency Temporary Standard (ETS) on formaldehyde.

As reported in the latest issue of "Lifelines," recent animal studies have shown an increased risk of nasal cancers from formaldehyde exposure at levels comparable to those in many working environments. So significant is the risk that top scientists have called for regulating formaldehyde as a cancer-causing substance.

The labor petition for an ETS asks OHSA to immediately take steps to reduce formaldehyde levels to the lowest feasible levels attainable by engineering control methods, a request that confronts directly OSHA's new policy of making personal protective equipment a primary means of controlling toxic exposures.

The petition also asks OSHA to include in its Formaldehyde ETS the following specific worker protections:

• In workplaces with potential exposure to formaldehyde, a determination of which employees are exposed and at what levels;

• Provision of all formaldehyde monitoring results to affected employees;

• Labeling of all formaldehyde containers with complete trade and generic chemical names.

• Provision by employer of respirators and appropriate personal protective clothing and equipment to exposed employees and the establishment of a respiratory protection program;

• Provision by employer of appropriate medical exams within 30 days of effective date of the ETS;

• Medical removal protection (rate retention) for any employee removed from exposure or limited as a result of medical exam results;

• Identification, upon request by OSHA, of all measures currently in effect to control worker exposure to formaldehyde, including any process, engineering, ventilation, administrative or product substitution measures, and documentation of exposure levels achieved by these means;

• An educational and training program for all employees at risk of exposure to formaldehyde.

In joining the Formaldehyde ETS petition, OCAW President Robert Goss noted the widespread use of formaldehyde at OCAW-represented workplaces. OCAW members produce formaldehyde and many thousands others use it in a variety of industries including resin production, pharmaceuticals, explosives, inks and cosmetics.

The chart on this page shows OCAW-represented plants known to produce or use formaldehyde extensively in resin production.

In addition to OCAW and the UAW, the following unions are also cosigners to the Formaldehyde petition: Allied Industrial Workers of America, Amalgamated Clothing and Textile Workers Union, AFL-CIO, American Federation of State, County and Municipal Employees, AFL-CIO Industrial Union Department, International Association of Machinists and Aerospace Workers, International Chemical Workers, International Molders and Allied Workers Union, United Brotherhood of Carpenters and Joiners of America, United Paperworkers International Union, United Rubber Workers of America, United Steelworkers of America.

Comp and Formaldehyde

A 34-year-old drywall finisher has been awarded worker compensation for pericarditis. resulting from exposure to formaldehyde.

Pericarditis, an inflammation of the sac surrounding the heart, is not usually associated with formaldehyde exposure.

The worker first saw a physician in 1979 complaining of shortness of breath and chest pain, which he contended was caused by exposure and inhalation of urea formaldehyde insulation at job sites where he went to drywall-finish.

After the insurance carrier denied the employee's claim for compensation, he submitted the claim to the State Industrial Commission on the basis of the formaldehyde exposure.

Although expert testimony was conflicting, one expert on formaldehyde foam insulation testified that it was quite possible for workers to become sensitized to the gas. In winter, the problem would be worse because doors and windows are shut and the heat is turned up.

Despite the conflicts in testimony, the State Industrial Commission awarded compensation to the employee and said he was entitled to medical, surgical and hospital benefits dating from his first visit to the physician in 1979.

The award is believed to be the first compensation case involving formaldehyde and pericarditis.

Local	Company	Location	No. of OCAW members	Use
1-793	Reichhold	White City, Ore.	20	primary producers
5-713	Hercules	Louisiana, Mo.	235	primary producers
8-397	Tenneco	Fords, N.J.	10	primary producers
8-566	Tenneco	Garfield, N.J.	110	primary producers
6-418	3-M	Cottage Grove, Mn.	602	phenol/formaldehyde resins
7-108	Reichhold	Ferndale, Mi.	203	phenol/formaldehyde resins
7-220	American Cyanamid	Kalamazoo, Mi.	50	melamine/formaldehyde
8-209	Reichhold	Niagara Falls, N.Y.	63	mel. and urea/formaldehyde
8-366	Reichhold	Andover, Mass.	38	mel. & urea/formaldehyde
8-891	Union Carbide	Bound Brook	541	phenol/formaldehyde resins
8-5370	American Cyanamid	Wallingford, Ct.	42	melamine/formaldehyde resins

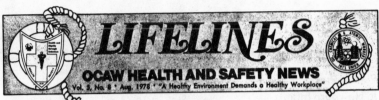

OCAW HEALTH AND SAFETY NEWS
Vol. 5, No. 8 · Aug. 1978 · "A Healthy Environment Demands a Healthy Workplace"

Ethylene Oxide Linked with Excess Leukemia Risk

Results of a recent Swedish study show a strong link between ethylene oxide exposure and leukemia, a cancer of the blood-forming system.

Three out of 100 workers in an ethylene oxide unit in Sweden were found suffering from leukemia, a 200 percent increase over the expected leukemia rate in the general population.

OCAW membes in four locations produce more than 20 percent of the total U.S. annual ethlyene oxide output. An Alert outlining the cancer threat as well as other vital information on ethylene oxide has been sent to the locals involved in primary production.

The affected groups include the workers at Jefferson Chemical, members of Port Neches, TX, Local 4-228; Houston Chemical, Beaumont, TX Local 4-243; Sunolin Chemical, Claymont, Delaware Local 8-930; and workers at BASF Wyandotte, Geismar, La. Local 4-620.

Ethylene oxide has widespead industrial use as a food and textile fumigant, an agricultural fungicide, and for sterilizing surgical instruments. It is also used as an intermediate in the production of ethylene glycol, polyglycols, glycol ethers, and esters, ethanolamines, acrylonitrile, plastics and surface-active agents.

There have been no studies published in the U.S. of mortality or causes of death among ethylene oxide workers. However, short-term tests on bacteria show the chemical to be a mutagen, causing changes in the hereditary material of living cells. More than 90 percent of the time, a chemical causing mutations will also cause cancer.

European animal studies add futher proof of ethylene oxide's cancer-causing potential. Animals exposed to 50 parts of ethylene oxide per million parts of air (ppm), the current OSHA 8-hour exposure limit, developed abnormalities of the chromosomes in the bone marrow.

Swedish chromosome studies of worker populations indicated chromosome damage at levels as low as one ppm ethylene oxide in workers exposed for approximately 15 years.

With local union and workman's committee cooperation, OCAW has requested OSHA's Cancer Identification Office to conduct chromosome and other biological tests on OCAW membes working in Ethylene Oxide production at Jefferson Chemicals, Local 4-228. These tests will show whether the workers are being affected by exposure to ethylene oxide.

Jefferson Chemical has been producing ethylene oxide for the last 25 years and there have been anecdotal reports of a number of deaths from Hodgkins Disease and leukemia.

Jefferson Chemicals, a subsidiary of Texaco, is located in Jefferson County, Texas, which has one of the highest rates of leukemia in the country, according to the National Cancer Institute's Atlas of Cancer Mortality for U.S. Counties, 1950-1969.

In fact, more than 75 percent of total U.S. ethylene oxide production is located in two states with high leukemia rates: Texas and Louisiana. Three of the four OCAW units producing ethylene oxide are located in the two states.

The National Cancer Institute is curently analyzing the causes of the more than 3,700 deaths in Texas recorded by the OCAW Membership Dept. between the years 1947-1977. This analysis might shed further light on the excess leukemia incidence in Texas and Louisiana.

Other Hazards

Aside fom its cancer-causing properties, ethylene oxide is also highly explosive, an eye and skin iritant and depressant to the central nervous system. The symptoms of chronic poisoning would be vague, such as: headaches, insomnia, irritability and an overall feeling of weakness

Exposure to high levels of ethylene oxide can cause respiratory irritation and a disease called pulmonary edema, in which your lungs fill with fluid.

Locals who plan to file OSHA complaints on ethylene oxide should use the General Duty Clause rather than the exposure limit of 50 ppm for an 8-hour average. If you file an OSHA complaint, you should do so through Steve Wodka, International Rep. in the Citizenship-Legislative Dept. This will speed up responses to your complaint and the International will assist you through all the phases of the inspection and follow-up.

If you work with ethylene oxide and do not receive an Alert from Vice-President Anthony Mazzocchi, please write his office for copies. There are potentially 30,000 OCAW workers at risk of exposure and Alerts will not reach everyone at risk. Check the list of jobs on this page to see if your occupation carries a risk of ethylene oxide exposue.

Jobs With Ethylene Oxide Risk

Acrylonitrile makers
Butyl cellosolve makers
Detergent makers
Disinfectant makers
Ethanolamine makers
Ethylene glycol makers
Exterminators
Foodstuff fumigators
Fumigant makers

Fungicide workers
Gasoline sweeteners
Grain elevator workers
Organic chemical synthesizers
Polyglycol makers
Polyoxirane makers
Rocket fuel handlers
Surfactant makers
Textile fumigators

Source: "Occupational Diseases, A Guide to Their Recognition," NIOSH Pub. No. 77-181, 1977.

The Plastic Age—An Age of Plastic Perils?

Almost everywhere we turn we are surrounded by plastic. Its uses and production are increasing everyday. As time passes we are becoming increasingly aware of some of the dangers that may resulting from such widespread use, often without adequate protection for workers and the public. Below are some recent examples.

Plastic Products Seen In Newborn Infants

A possible new danger arising from the use of plastics in medical procedures has been reported by researchers at Washington University (*N. Engl. J.,* 2/20/75).

The plasticizers, which are used to make vinyl plastics pliant, can be leached out of the plastics by blood. They have been found in tissues and organs of patients receiving transfusions, plastics catheters and tubes.

The present study found high levels of the plasticizer DEHP in various tissues of newborn infants who died at birth or shortly thereafter. In those infants dying of *necrotizing enterocolitis,* a common premature infant gut disease, significant levels of DEHP were found in the gut.

At this point, however, it is impossible to determine whether the high levels resulted from an already weak organ or whether they contributed to the further weakening.

Although DEHP has not been found to be directly toxic it is thought to affect activity of the blood circulatory system and to be toxic to rapidly growing cells. It is also unclear whether DEHP passes from a pregnant mother to an unborn child but it has been shown to cause birth defects in animal studies.

DEHP is found throughout the adult and child population, probably resulting from such environmental sources as plastic food bags. The long-range meaning of this is not clear as yet. However, in studies of beef heart, as much as 60 percent of the fat found was attributed to DEHP. If true in humans, this may have an effect on the heart attack rate.

PVC Safety Increasing

Now that the legal stumbling blocks have been hurdled, the new vinyl chloride standard goes into effect April 1, 1975. And suddenly new technology has been springing forth.

Just a few years ago workers who were tank cleaners manually chipped away at vinyl chloride tanks between batches. Now a small enclosed reactor is nearing design completion. Alarm systems sensitive to 1 ppm are rapidly entering the market.

PLASTICS CAN DECOMPOSE INTO TOXIC SUBSTANCES

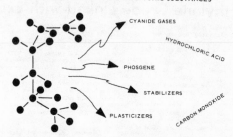

CYANIDE GASES
HYDROCHLORIC ACID
PHOSGENE
STABILIZERS
PLASTICIZERS
CARBON MONOXIDE

Plastics are made of long molecules called polymers and other substances such as plasticizers, stabilizers, dyes, fillers, etc., to give them different colors, shapes and properties. When exposed to the elements, chemicals, heated, burned, etc., plastics decompose, often yielding toxic, even deadly substances, endangering both workers and the public.

Warning! Plastics Fumes May Be Deadly

Plastics are highly flammable. When burned, they give off gases and other substances which are dangerous and can be deadly.

Firefighters Study

A study of the entire Boston Fire Dept. showed a loss in pulmonary function of *more than twice* what would normally be expected in such a group. Researchers at the Harvard School of Public Health conducted lung function studies of the firefighters during 1970-72.

The firefighters showed a rate of loss in lung function which equaled that of patients with chronic obstructive lung disease. The study will continue with a focus on identification of the most hazardous exposures and air sampling to determine products formed in the combustion process.

Wrapping Meat Hazardous

"Meat wrappers asthma" is a "modern" disease resulting from plastic exposure. (See January, 1974 "Lifelines" for discussion.) Heat-activated labels are now reported as the major cause of the disease which is marked by sneezing, nasal congestion, coughs and asthmatic responses. When the labels are heated, they emit organic copolymer fumes. Nine out of 13 persons exposed to these fumes developed breathing problems within minutes.

An even more alarming development is a recent study of rats exposed to fumes from the combustion of fire-retarded polyurethane foam.

Burning Foam Toxic

Scientists at the University of Utah's Flammability Research Center discovered that the fumes caused grand mal or severe epileptic seizures and were fatal to exposed rats. The rats' behavior was also severely impaired, and resembled the behavior of humans after smoke intoxication.

Upon analysis, a phosphate compound was found in the fumes which has been proven toxic at levels lower than one part per million! Clearly, more research is needed to weigh the risks versus the benefits of fire-retardant materials, as well as to assess the risks plastics pose when burned.

A step in the right direction is a recent consent agreement between the Federal Trade Commission, the Society of the Plastics Industry, and the 25 major manufacturers of foamed plastics to label these materials. The labels will now carry a "Warning! This product is highly flammable" designation. The agreement also provides for a $5 million research program to study the flammability of foamed or cellular plastic products.

The principal would-be protective agency on occupational health in the government is the Occupational Safety and Health Administration (OSHA), set up in 1971 following passage of the Occupational Safety and Health Act.

The Reagan administration appointed as administrator of OSHA Thorne Auchter, formerly executive vice president of Auchter Construction of Jacksonville, Florida—cited by OSHA 48 separate times for violations of the Occupational Safety and Health Act before Auchter took over supervising the handling of the Occupational Safety and Health Act.

"It's unfair to characterize his company's record as bad," insists Foster James, director of information for OSHA. "Only one or two of the situations were serious."

Meanwhile, OSHA has been making drastic cutbacks in enforcement. Comparing 1981 to 1980, citations for "willfull" violations were down 75%, citations for what are considered "serious" violations were reduced by 32%, the number of penalties imposed was lowered by 48% and the dollar amount of penalties was down 54%.

Under Auchter, OSHA procedures have been substantially changed: a complaint to OSHA may now only be made by employees in writing and only those involving "imminent danger" are to be checked out by an OSHA inspector. Employers are now able to come into "compliance" by voluntarily abating the hazard and no OSHA inspection is required to determine that this was actually done.

Dr. Rafael Moure is the industrial hygienist for the Oil, Chemical & Atomic Workers International Union.

Says Moure: "What is happening with this administration is that they want to turn the clock back 15 years when we didn't have the Occupational Safety and Health Act. Basically the mandate that Auchter has received from Reagan has been to stop the agency from being an effective agency that is going to enforce the law."

Under Auchter, he says, OSHA has not developed any new standards but has emphasized reduction of existing standards. "For example, we put in a tremendous amount of time and energy getting the agency to pass a standard on access to medical records. Now, they are reducing the scope of this standard by seeing that fewer workers have the right to obtain their medical records."

Rather than conducting investigations and developing records for people exposed to the substances that are on the Registry of Toxic Substances," continues Moure, OSHA now says, "No, we don't want records to be kept and be available to workers on all those substances, around 30,000; we would like to reduce that to 3,500."

The inspection staff has been cut from 1,600 to 1,000; inspections are way down, there "are hardly any" follow-up inspections.

"And all down the line there is an attempt—just simply because it is easier and cheaper for industry—to water down the standards," he says.

OSHA, he goes on, is supposed to be in government "the advocate of workers for occupational health." The philosophy of the Occupational Safety and Health Act was to "tell the workers, 'Look, you don't have to subsidize industry with your health anymore.' "

Auchter's "only claim to fame as far as occupational health is that in a period of seven years his company was cited fourteen times by OSHA and in addition to that he was an organizer of Youths for Reagan and a big fundraiser in the Florida area," says Moure. "So that's how he got the job."

And OSHA has become "just like the EPA" under Reagan, says Moure. Auchter is "basically a political hack and his job is to basically wreck the agency, water down the standards and to use every possible device with the people that are working for him to water down this law and to make this law ineffective.

"What they're trying to do now is to destroy OSHA—the same way with the Environmental Protection Agency."

And the health of workers, Moure concludes, "is suffering today."

Workers in the chemical industry are particularly affected.

The Council on Economic Priorities, a New York-based organization which does research on the practices of U.S. corporations reported in a 1981 study, *Occupational Safety and Health in the Chemical Industry,* that through the years the chemical industry has had a rate of violations per OSHA inspection nearly three times the national industrial average.

The group "found the chemical industry to be among the most hazardous in the nation" and in "number of serious violations it exceeded all other industries except mining."

Dupont ranked "as the most problematic of the large chemical companies" not only in initial violations but in "willful violations"—defined as "a situation where the employer was aware that a hazardous condition existed and made no reasonable effort to eliminate the hazard." Over 30% of the instances of willful violations in the entire chemical industry between 1972 and 1979 involved Dupont, the council reported.

In its "profile" of the chemical companies and the hazards their workers have undergone, the council said there have been "major safety and health problems at Dupont plants in Deepwater, New Jersey and Chicago. Contamination of drinking water at the Belle, West Virginia plant led to liver and eye cancers and other health effects. Worker exposure to known and suspected carcinogens such as benzidine, moca and acrylonitrile has also been cause for concern." Dupont lists 134,200 employees.

The Allied Corporation, with 49,014 workers, was ranked just above Dupont and the council said "the company's Moundsville, West Virginia plant had the dubious distinction of receiving the first OSHA citation for exposures to mercury 'likely to cause death or serious physical harm to employees.' A retrospective study of workers at an Allied plant in Buffalo, New York who had worked with benzidene and other potential carcinogens, showed that 115 of them had developed bladder tumors. Problems have also cropped up at Allied plants in Baton Rouge, Louisiana and Danville, Illinois. The most notorious of Allied's health hazards was Kepone, produced by what was then its Life Sciences Products affiliate. The chemical caused sterility and nervous disorders in 75 employees in the mid-1970's and seriously polluted the James River in Virginia."

The best of the bad was Union Carbide, with 115,763 employees, and its record is ugly. The council noted that "the brain cancer deaths of 16 workers at Union Carbide's Texas City, Texas plant has caused substantial concern" and " of the 63 cases of angiosarcoma, a liver cancer, worldwide, six were

employees of Carbide's South Charleston plant, which produces 400 chemicals including vinyl chloride. Vinyl chloride
workers at the plant were found to have four times the expected incidence of leukemia in 1976 and twice the expected
incidence of brain cancer."

* * *

"Farmers: All across the nation today the conditions are
fine for spraying," said the weatherman on an all-weather
cable television channel.

And that day in 1982, as on many days, America became
saturated with agricultural sprays. A ride through much of
American farmland has become a rural version of driving the
Jersey Turnpike through industrial New Jersey: the acrid,
piercing, foul smell of chemical sprays pervade.

As Friends of the Earth reported in a 1981 *Status Report on
Pesticides:*

> Last Year, Americans used well over a billion pounds of
> chemical pesticides and herbicides. We are all served up a
> stew of chemical leftovers as residues of these pesticides
> and the compounds to which they degrade find their way
> into our food and water. Sometimes we are exposed di-
> rectly, as when residents of farming communities are struck
> by drifting pesticide spray or children play in city parks that
> have just been treated with herbicides.
>
> The effect of these substances on our health, not to men-
> tion the health of our environment, is not completely
> known. In fact, our government approved many of the pes-
> ticides now in use without any information on the damage
> which chronic exposure might cause humans. Actual cause
> is often difficult to pinpoint, but medical case histories have
> established links between such problems as chloracne, ner-
> vous system disorders, cancer, abnormal pregnancies, or
> declining sperm counts and exposure to one or more of
> these poorly tested chemicals. For some, this is a matter of

"acceptable risk." For others, it's a matter of temporary illness or permanent health disorders!

Chemical herbicides and insecticides are among the compounds commonly classified as pesticides. These pesticides are applied to farm lands, timber stands, and highway, railroad, and powerline rights-of-way. They are used to kill unwanted pests, both weeds or insects. Many of these chemicals were developed for use during wartime. Since World War II the production of toxic pesticides has doubled every nine years to reach a staggering total of 1.6 *BILLION* pounds in 1980. Many of the most hazardous of these poisons have been banned, but are still produced in the United States for export. They return to haunt our dinner tables as residues contained in imported fruits and vegetables.

While our government has designed programs to ensure that we are protected from harmful or carelessly used pesticides, pressure from the chemical industry generally has ensured that these programs are too weak to do an adequate job. New pesticides are introduced before the government can adequately evaluate them. The pesticide maufacturers claim they test the safety of their products, but it is rare that they go to the expense of performing exhaustive tests. Federal agencies lack either the will or the clout to demand adequate safety tests. Proof exists that poorly tested chemicals enter the market. Furthermore, potentially harmful pesticides that were approved years ago, when less stringent health testing requirements were in force, remain on the market, despite their inability to meet the new testing standards.

"The federal government has abdicated its responsibility to protect citizens from involuntary exposure to harmful pesticides," declared Friends of the Earth, which said "our best hope is to turn to the states for protection." (That's why the chemical industry has been moving to prohibit states from enacting regulations on pesticides.)

Friends of the Earth noted: "Wind-blown pesticides reach our lakes and streams and leach into underground aquifers, and massive road-side weed abatement programs blast unsuspecting home-owners with harmful defoliants. As much as 70 percent of aerially applied pesticides drift off target."

Said the group:

> In 1979 FOE petitioned the EPA and the Federal Aviation Administration to set federal regulatory standards for applying restricted chemicals—both on the ground and from the air. We asked for the creation of buffer zones of 1500 feet for applications by air and 500 feet for applications on the ground between the land to be sprayed and other privately owned property. Requirements that prior notification of spraying plans be given to owners within this zone and that insurance be carried by sprayers to cover the claims of those who suffered medical problems or property loss from improperly applied chemical pesticide were also sought. Although the petitions were published in the Federal Register and public comment was invited, NO ACTION has been taken in more than two years. With the new administration's support of the pesticide industry, none is expected.

Cancer has become a principal harvest of farmers and farmworkers who use chemical pesticides, herbicides and fertilizers. In some agricultural areas they call it "farmers' cancer."

"EPA provides virtually no protection at all," Charles Horwitz of the Migrant Legal Action Program told a 1978 conference on "Pesticides and Human Health" conducted by the Society for Occupational and Environmental Health in Washington, D.C.

He spoke of a total of five million farmworkers in America, consisting of 1.2 million migrant farmworkers and 3.8 million seasonal farmworkers, as well as thousands of crop dusting pilots and many thousands of neighbors, rural residents and automobile drivers who pass through irrigated fields where there is pesticide exposure and through fields where there are crop dusting airplanes. Thus, perhaps ten million people are affected by pesticide poisoning abuse in rural areas and this does not include consumers."

Farmworkers are especially affected, having to go from farm to farm "sometimes ten or fifteen farms in the course of a year and we believe that at least once a year, and maybe twice or three times a year, they are exposed to toxic pesticides," said Horwitz. "Farmworkers are exposed to pesticides even before they are born since pesticide residues have been found to pass from mother to fetus in utero. Farmworker children, even before they are old enough to work, are exposed to pesticide poisoning because they live near farms and migrant housing camps which are very often sprayed with pesticide residue drifts from crop dusting airplanes."

Compared to the average life expectancy of 70 in America, farmworkers have a life expectancy of 41, he noted.

And he hit on how the EPA "under pressure from agribusinesses shows more sympathy for the perpetuators" of pesticide poisonings "than for the victims."

In 1979, this legal action was brought before the EPA by the National Association of Farmworkers Organizations, the Illinois Migrant Council and three farmworkers doused with the pesticide Carbaryl sprayed from an airplane while they were harvesting asparagus:

BEFORE THE UNITED STATES
ENVIRONMENTAL PROTECTION AGENCY

In the Matter of an Effective)   Docket No.
Pesticide Incident Reporting)
System)
)
_____)

I.   INTRODUCTION

This is a petition to the United States Environmental Protection Agency (hereafter EPA) to protect farmworkers from work-related pesticide injuries. Towards this end petitioners request that EPA adopt a mandatory pesticide incident reporting system, initiate a comprehensive demonstration monitoring project, require new labelling instructions on all registered pesticide products, and provide funds to educate farmworkers about pesticide hazards. The petition is submitted pursuant to the Federal Insecticide, Fungicide and Rodenticide Act (hereafter FIFRA), 7 U.S.C. § 136w(a) and the Administrative Procedure Act, 5 U.S.C. § 553(e) and 555(e).

The action noted that the "EPA has a legal mandate to effectively monitor, implement and manage" the system of registering pesticides, under the Federal Insecticide, Fungicide and Rodenticide Act (FIFRA).

It went on:

> Any major decision in the registration process must be based on a determination of whether there will be "any unreasonable adverse effects on the environment" resulting from the use of the pesticide. The statute defines this standard as "any unreasonable risk to man or the environment, taking into account the economic, social, and environmental costs and benefits of the use of any pesticide." Thus, registration of a pesticide must be denied when unreasonable adverse effects to man or the environment are found; if a pesticide is registered for general use and later adverse effects are found, the product must be reclassified for restricted use, suspended or cancelled. A determination of adverse effects requires a monitoring system that measures the impact of pesticides on human beings.

FIFRA's Legislative History Also Mandates An Effective Monitoring System

FIFRA's legislative history also supports the assertion that Congress intended a strong human effects monitoring system. The monitoring provision of FIFRA, like that of the enforcement and registration provisions, was "designed to provide for tighter control of pesticide registration and to insure protection to man and to the environment." In fact, in 1972 Congress adopted the monitoring provision precisely because a Presidential Scientific Advisory Commission concluded that the "monitoring programs, to obtain systematic data on pesticide residues, should be expanded." In 1978 Congress gave still more human effects monitoring responsibilities to the EPA.

Farmworkers are often Severely Harmed by Pesticide Misuse

Over five million farmworkers labor in agriculture each year in the United States. When they are in fields they frequently are exposed to pesticides by airplane overspray and by dust, soil and crops laden with pesticides. Since neither protective clothing nor water to wash their hands is generally supplied, these workers often eat their lunch and drink water with hands containing pesticide residue. In addition, clothing has been found to catch and retain pesticide residues, greatly increasing the possibility of dermal absorption of chemical residues by farmworkers.

The action cited "in addition to those injuries to farmworker petitioners," these "typical examples of agricultural poisoning incidents:"

- On March 12, 1979, a farmworker in Homestead, Florida was sprayed with pesticides by a cropdusting airplane and by a field applicator while loading tomatoes. He suffered sores and lesions all over his body and had severe eye problems.
- In early March, 1979, about 25 farmworkers in Collier County, Florida were sprayed with nitrogen by a cropdusting airplane and suffered sores and skin irritations.
- Seven farmworkers near Pandoro, Ohio were deliberately sprayed with Ethephon (Ethrel) while they were picketing at a tomato farm on August 28, 1978. One worker suffered chest pains and has been unable to work for six months.
- During August, 1978, Toxaphene and Orthene sprayed by a cropdusting airplane drifted over a state labor camp near Modesto, California causing nausea, stomach aches, headaches, and eye problems to 14 farmworker children.
- In June, 1978, near Alton, Colorado, five farmworkers were sprayed with Toxaphene and Parathion by a cropdusting airplane, causing them nausea and headaches.
- In June, 1978, farmworkers near Grand Rapids, Michigan, suffered sores, breathing difficulties and lung congestion arising from the spraying of Captan.
- Seven farmworkers were sprayed with Difolatan in fields near Immokalee, Florida in January, 1978. They suffered large sores on their hands for several weeks.
- Twelve farmworkers were sprayed in April, 1978 with pesticides by a cropdusting airplane near Edinburg, Texas causing them skin rashes and breathing difficulties.
- In mid-June, 1976, farmworkers and their children in Berrien, Cass and Van Buren counties, Michigan were ex-

posed to Captan and Benlate and suffered severe skin rashes.

- A California farmworker pesticide applicator died in December, 1976 after suffering swelling and pains in his mouth and face after a leak in a tractor hose and valve sprayed Telone onto his face.

The EPA rejected the petition in 1982.

In 1980, the National Rural Health Council held a series of forums around the U.S. entitled: "Pesticide Use and Misuse: Farmworkers and Small Farmers Speak on the Problem."

In Pharr, Texas, Ocoee, Florida and Salinas, California, farmers and farmworkers told of instances—hundreds upon hundreds of instances—of pesticide exposure leading to blindness, chronic headaches, permanent disability, cancer and death. And there was complaint after complaint of a general lack of information about the dangers of pesticides and government collaboration with the producers of poison.

At Ocoee, farmworker Francisco Rodriguez, after speaking of health problems he and farmworkers he knew had been suffering, pleaded for "enforcement of these laws against pesticides, because we are not the only ones that can get harmed. We are the laborers. Also the consumer is harmed. Some lettuce, some tomatoes, and other things that have pesticides, are harmful and we don't want to harm our brothers."

Farmworker Paula Rivera said: "One time there was a bunch of little kids playing with a pesticide can, and it had been raining, and the children they don't know very much, and they were playing in this, and I don't know how it happened, probably the child drank the water, and a few hours later she died. And I would want everybody here to open their ears and their eyes and see what really is happening to many people, and I wish that someone would do something about it."

John Traunfeld, at Ocoee, a former Cooperative Extension employee who left to manage a vegetable cooperative, said farmers did not have access to accurate information on pesticides—from application procedures to disposal methods to health hazards. He spoke of farmers becoming dependent on pesticides by not being involved in crop rotation and diversification to control insect growth and fungus. He said insufficient research was being conducted into "integrated pest management"—a mixed approach to deal with insects—and that chemical companies are not receptive to integrated pest management because they suspect it would be difficult for them to make money on it. He called on farmers "to begin asking hard questions about the kind of agricultural economy which is unable to offer us a decent living along with a safe environment for us all." He concluded, "People have created the present situation and people can change it."

In Salinas, Paul Barnett of the California Agrarian Action Project hit at land grant universities being co-opted through chemical company funding. Chemical companies give more than 400 grants a year to the University of California alone, he said. And, Barnett charged, the chemical industry provides people who are supposed to be independent researchers with inducements like paid vacations, liquor and consulting fees. Such supposed agricultural experts end up recommending pesticides, often by brand names used by their benefactors. He declared that EPA has often relied on fraudulent data from manufacturers about pesticides and didn't enforce the law in any case.

And Jessie Delacruz, the first woman organizer of the United Farmworkers of California, said, "I want to see, I want to live long enough to see my great grandchildren, and I don't want any harm for them. I don't want them born deformed because of the chemicals and the pesticides."

"We give this testimony and we give it with our hearts," said farmworker Guadalupe Hernandez in Pharr, "and we want these laws enforced. You are playing with our children's lives, and the lives of our fellow workers, and you need to do something to remedy the situation. Don't just say you are going to do something, and then forget about it the next day. Do it. We want to see it done."

Or as Bruce Hawley, assistant director of the American Farm Bureau Federation's Washington office, told a hearing of the House Subcommittee on Department Operations, Research and Foreign Agriculture in 1981: "Farm Bureau members buy, store and apply pesticides, have front-line exposure to whatever risks are involved with chemical handling and use, and expect the federal government to fulfill its responsibility of evaluating pesticide safety and effectiveness.

"EPA has let us down," declared Hawley. "We believe EPA's record is one of failure to protect farmers, ranchers and other users, the public and the environment."

Health professionals are also extremely concerned. Thomas P. Butcher, Jr., clinical coordinator of the Acadania Emergency Rural Systems Council in Lousiana, wrote in a 1981 letter to the EPA: "We are experiencing a serious public health problem from current pesticide and herbicide use.

"Our overall cancer mortality rates in the rural Acadiana parishes far exceed the national average and the rates for the petro-chemical corridor along the Mississippi River between Baton Rouge and New Orleans. Since we lack pollutant sources such as chemical plants, urban congestion, etc., agrichemical induced carcinogenisis should be suspected . . . The greater the percentage of the population living in rural areas in a particular parish, the higher the cancer rate is.

"Overall, I feel the Department of Agriculture should begin to research and disseminate information about alternatives to agrichemicals, i.e. integrated pest management. A survey of publications at my local county agent's office revealed repeatedly, for each crop, farmers are advised to use dangerous, toxic chemicals for pests and weeds, with no mention of prevention or safer, non-chemical routes to the same goal, and without mention that these should be used only when a problem is definitely present. The herbicide ads on the local media, for example, repeatedly advocate chemical use prophylactically, without waiting to see if a weed problem really exists. Similarly, the county agent's corn growing brochure advocates 2,4-D application without even attempting cultivation or other known weed control procedures. Recently, a Hammond, Louisiana man died after splashing a small amount of 2,4-D on his groin, yet local agriculture officials have little advice they can offer farmers regarding weeds or pests that does not involve exposing them to extremely toxic chemicals."

Documentation of the link between chemical pesticides, herbicides and fertilizers and cancer continues to grow.

A 1971 *American Journal of Epidemiology* study found a "significant association between farming occupations and death from leukemia and multiple myeloma."

AMERICAN JOURNAL OF EPIDEMIOLOGY
Copyright © 1971 by The Johns Hopkins University

Vol. 94, No. 4
Printed in U.S.A.

ORIGINAL CONTRIBUTIONS

LEUKEMIA AND MULTIPLE MYELOMA IN FARMERS

SAMUEL MILHAM, JR.[1]

(Received for publication March 5, 1971)

Milham, S., Jr. (Washington State Department of Social and Health Services, Division of Health, Olympia Airport, Olympia, Washington 98501). Leukemia and multiple myeloma in farmers. *Amer J Epidem* 94: 307–310, 1971.—Analysis of deaths from leukemia-lymphoma group cancers and occupation as stated on death certificates revealed a statistically significant association between farming occupations and death from leukemia and multiple myeloma. No such association was seen for Hodgkin's disease, reticulum cell sarcoma, or other lymphomas. The leukemia-farming association was strongest in men under age 60 with lymphatic and acute types of leukemia. Poultry farmers showed the highest proportionate case excess in the leukemia study. These findings are consistent with the hypothesis that agricultural environments contain agents which may cause leukemia.

leukemia; lymphoma; multiple myeloma

These findings are consistent with the hypothesis that agricultural environments contain agents which may cause leukemia.

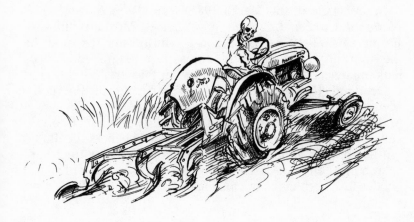

This report from a 1979 issue of the *American Journal of Epidemiology* again noted a high incidence of leukemia among farmers.

AMERICAN JOURNAL OF EPIDEMIOLOGY
Copyright © 1979 by The Johns Hopkins University School of Hygiene and Public Health
All rights reserved

Vol. 110, No. 3
Printed in U.S.A.

LEUKEMIA AMONG NEBRASKA FARMERS: A DEATH CERTIFICATE STUDY[1]

AARON BLAIR AND TERRY L. THOMAS

A. Blair (Environmental Epidemiology Branch, National Cancer Institute, 3C07 Landow Bldg., Bethesda, MD 20205), and T. L. Thomas. Leukemia among Nebraska farmers: A death certificate study. *Am J Epidemiol* 110:264–273, 1979.

The risk of leukemia among farmers was studied using records of death certificates from Nebraska, 1957–1974. Comparison of occupation, as recorded on the death certificate, for 1084 leukemia deaths and 2168 deaths from other causes, matched for age at death, year of death, county of residence, race, and sex, revealed an elevated risk of leukemia among farmers (odds ratio = 1.25). The risk was greatest among farmers born after 1900 and dying before age 66 (odds ratio = 1.83). Stratification by county of residence showed a significantly elevated risk for farmers from heavy corn producing counties.

agricultural workers' diseases; death certificates; leukemia; mortality

It noted that farmers are exposed to "leukemogenic agents" and said "the risk of leukemia was increased among farmers born after, but not before, 1900, suggesting a relationship with agricultural exposures of recent origin."

In an article in the March 1981 issue of the *Journal of the National Cancer Institute,* on "Cancer Mortality in Iowa Farmers, 1971–1978," Dr. Leon F. Burmeister reported that the mortality rate for lip, stomach, prostate cancer and leukemia were "significantly higher for farmers."

Declared Burmeister, of the Department of Preventive Medicine and Environmental Health of the College of Medicine of the University of Iowa: "This study is one of several that indicate that some aspects of farmers' health are not as good as generally believed." He called for further research into "the possible roles of fertilizers, insecticides, fungicides and herbicides in causing cancer."

And cancer is not the only consequence.

A 1980 study of children of Imperial Valley, California farmworkers showed they were born with shortened or missing limbs—birth defects—at a rate 13 times that of newborns nationwide, and pesticides were pointed to as the cause.

Some 2,514 births over a four year period were studied by Dr. David Schwartz, an internist at Boston City Hospital, Dr. Ruth Heifetz, a professor of occupational medicine at the University of California at San Diego and Linda Newsum, a medical sociologist. "The offspring where one or both parents were agricultural workers were found to have a prevalance rate of 5.2 limb reduction—defined as a shortening or deleted portion of a limb—defects per 1,000 live births," said the study, while the rate per 1,000 births for such birth defects in the western U.S. is .4.

The conclusion of the National Science Foundation-supported research was that "the results of our study further implicate pesticides as a human teratogen."

Dr. Schwartz noted that "Imperial County uses the largest amount" of pesticides of any county in California. "Growers there use about three times the amount of pesticides that are used in other agricultural areas of the state." Further, "there are pesticide dumps throughut the county. Children swim and fish in canals which contain pesticide runoff."

***

People who live near waste dumps or polluting industries, employees of industries involved with toxic substances, and farmers and farmworkers in chemical agriculture, are on poison's front line—but indeed, we all are, too.

No Need to Grow Food with Poison

"Everything we grow on the farm we do without chemical pesticides, herbicides and fertilizers," Andy Snyder is saying amidst the rows of spinach, lettuce, potatoes, broccoli, tomatoes, cabbage, beans, turnips, onions, cucumbers, cauliflower, carrots, swiss chard, zucchini—and much more—all vigorous and bursting from the earth of his 125-acre farm nestled in the center of Vermont.

Why?

"Number one," says Snyder without hesitation, "it just makes sense."

While not busy growing and selling food, Snyder is president of the New England-based Natural Organic Farmers Association, a group which has attracted national and international attention.

"We are familiar with," Snyder says, "and blessed with the brains to know what the seed companies and the chemical companies are attempting to do." He speaks of seed companies "bought out left and right by chemical and pharmaceutical companies" and no longer particularly in "business to sell seeds. Burpee, for instance, is owned by ITT and you have companies like Purex and Kerr-McGee owning seed companies.

"Seeds are almost a loss leader. What they're in business doing is developing varieties which are absolutely dependent upon chemical pesticides, herbicides and fertilizers to grow well. That's the whole hybridizing process they are going through in their development of new seed."

47

Such seed would give the farmer no choice other than "using the pesticides, herbicides and chemical fertilizers that these seed varieties depend on" and that, says the Florence, Vermont farmer, "would be a real selling-out on our part.

"So we try to obtain seed that is not from these companies."

And Snyder's independence doesn't stop there. "It's honestly our belief," he is saying, "that we can grow a higher quality crop without using any of these things"—the synthetic pesticides, herbicides and fertilizers.

"The more each year you till the soil," he says with a warmth, a love of earth, the "more you get the feeling for the tilth" of a soil. "And if you're dependent on chemical fertilizers, your dependence increases each and every year. If that's the only fertilizer you're putting down—something out of a bag of 5-10-10 from Agway or whatever, the cellular structure, the molecular structure in the soil itself deteriorates—and it can be felt.

"This necessitates a greater and greater investment in chemical fertilizer if one wants to be able to grow a comparable crop year after year." A farmer thus becomes a junkie to the petrochemical-based fertilizer.

"That's not true when you farm organically, using what is available to you and going by the principle of returning to the soil as much as or more than you take," says Snyder. "That way you're developing the organic matter and the humus in the soil."

You are free of "outside fertilizer sources."

Compost is at the base of what Snyder calls a "balanced system" to raise a "quality crop, a crop that is not all water.

"If you take a look at some crops that get shipped in from California, broccoli for instance," Snyder is saying, "sometimes you can almost poke it with a fork and it will just ooze water. There's just no quality to it.

"We need to have and we demand from ourselves having the highest quality available," says Snyder of food from his farm, "and we're able to do that by organic fashion. And in some ways it's much more labor-intensive and in other ways it's much more expensive but at the same time the quality is there and people appreciate it; they really do."

Today "people want more control of their lives, particularly of what they take into their bodies, and I think people are trying to do things in a more natural fashion," he says. "And if we can help them do that in an honest way and give them something that tastes good at the same time and is good for them, we come home with a little more than just dollars in our pocket. We come home with a little bit of pride."

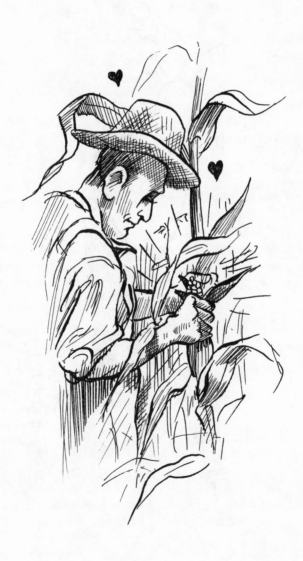

Chemical farming causes food to become bloated with water, soaked up in between shots of chemicals.

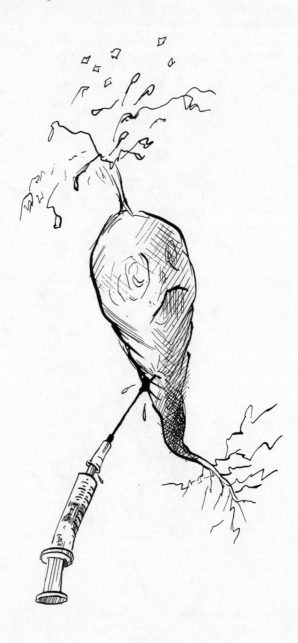

"Often you will see that the size of a crop might be larger if it's grown in a chemical fashion, sometimes to the point where like a mutant they will grow incredibly in short spans and will respond almost overnight to a pellet of nitrogen their roots finally come in contact with," he says. "They will grow an inordinate amount in a very short time and split. If it's a tomato it'll split. If it's a cabbage it'll split."

They are "using water to substitute for some of the nutrients which are in the soil which, if given a longer period of time in the soil, they would absorb," says Snyder. And thus such crops become cheapened, they do "not have the qualities of vitamins and minerals that organic produce does."

It is not just the conventional testing for acid and alkaline—Ph testing—that Snyder does for the earth on his farm. He tests for a wide variety of trace minerals, and adds minerals when called for. Also, in addition to compost he applies mixes of liquid seaweed and fish emulsion, spraying them on the leaves of plants.

Without herbicides killing weeds, he does his weeding with tiller, hoe and by hand. "And the amount of work that I do compared to a guy who goes out and sprays herbicides, it's night and day," Snyder admits. "But at the same time, he doesn't grow the quality of crops that I do."

Snyder's farm is rich with companion plantings to discourage insect pests. Basil surrounds the carrot beds, marigolds encircle broccoli and cauliflower, nasturtiums shelter zucchini. In the greenhouse, Snyder uses "beneficial insects" to go after damaging ones.

Pesticides "of an organic nature"—made of flowers and plants that repel certain bugs—are used by Snyder, and there is some handpicking of insect eggs from plants. He says "we control insects as well as any chemical farmer, but in a more organic approach."

Snyder says that if he were involved in chemical farming, he'd feel "guilt-ridden. I'm a bright enough guy to know that the quality would be compromised." And he feels certain of a link between food grown with chemicals and ill health.

He speaks of seeing "spectrograms of whole wheat bread compared to white bread and it's amazing to take a look at a white bread structure which is so broken, it almost looks like

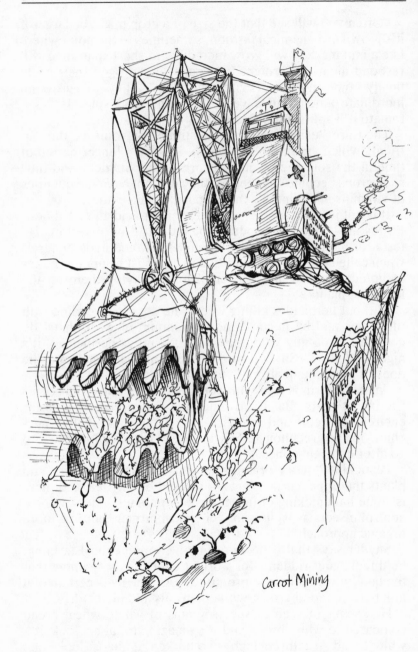

Carrot Mining

a destroyed cell, whereas you have this beautiful kaleidoscope effect from a spectrogram of whole wheat bread." He feels he knows "what looks healthy and what doesn't, and I really believe food raised in an organic fashion is much healthier. When I sell beans at the farmers' market, compared to some guy who's a chemical farmer, my beans shine—they've really got a glow, a healthy look to them."

The "environmental winds that blow over the agricultural community do absolutely create a tremendous health hazard to the consumer, not to mention the farmer," says Snyder. "There is the farmer out there breathing in herbicides and pesticides and fertilizers. My God, the cancer rate among chemical farmers is tremendous. That has to tell you something."

He feels it is thoroughly practical for farmers to get off the agrichemical fix and farm naturally.

"I think the economics of providing wholesome food grown organically is here," says Snyder, and he stresses that he doesn't mean "every farm having a couple of goats and a couple of chickens and people running around barefoot" but viable enterprises, broadly situated geographically, and providing food in "a well-rounded diversified fashion."

The key problem is that many farmers "are absolutely slaves to the chemical companies." Only in recent years with the price of the main ingredient of synthetic pesticides, herbicides and fertilizers—oil—skyrocketing has there been the realization that something is happening that "will absolutely spell the downfall" of chemical farming. To switch to organic methods is "more of a mental adjustment than it is anything else," he adds.

Whether or not farmers are all capable of making this change "remains to be seen," but if food production is not detoxified, disconnected from the chemical companies and the rising price of oil and reconnected to nature's balance, it is "going to mean a whole lot of hungry people in the world in a few years," declares the Vermont farmer.

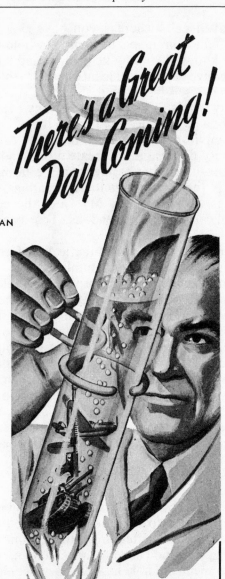

There's a Great Day Coming!

WAR-INSPIRED RESEARCH PROMISES
New Wonders **FOR THE FARM**

During War or Peace **DELCO APPLIANCES**
Do the Job Better

Out of War They Came

It was in the desperate cauldron of war, of World War II, that many of the poisons widely used in our time were concocted. American corporations and scientists joined with the government on chemical warfare research, a program paralleling the development of the atomic bomb.

In both endeavors, those involved sought after the war to spin off commercially what had been developed. Insects, for example, were used to test toxic gases being developed for war use, and so by 1945 those chemicals able to devastate particular insects were well known—and became the base of a huge postwar insect-killing industry.

The corporate/scientific/government chemical establishment that was assembled during World War II began engaging in an ultimate act of chemical warfare two decades later, in the Vietnam War. An ultra-toxic herbicide was rained down leaving an endless harvest of genetic defects and cancer; tens of millions of Vietnamese and 2.4 million American soldiers are estimated as having been contaminated with Agent Orange in Vietnam.

How those responsible have done this is a demonstration of the workings of the Poison Conspiracy.

The government and the major chemical companies which caused dioxin-laced Agent Orange to be showered with abandon on Vietnam have aggressively refused to accept responsibility for the widescale contamination they produced.

"The chemical companies' attitude is deny, deny, deny," says attorney Victor J. Yannacone, Jr., lead counsel for the lawyers representing the veterans exposed to Agent Orange in Vietnam. These veterans have been seeing their offspring born with genetic damage and they themselves are suffering and dying from awful maladies, especially cancer. The government, says Yannacone, has joined in a pattern of cover-up. He calls the Agent Orange situation "Orangegate."

But the poison of Agent Orange and how friends and foe were contaminated by it is not just a phenomenon of war.

Dioxin-laced poison—the same lethal toxin that was in Agent Orange—remains in wide use today, for weed control in rice fields and rangelands. Dioxin is in widely sold consumer products, too, including the popular Silvex herbicide for gardens.

Yannacone cites studies at the University of Wisconsin showing that just 50 parts *per trillion* of dioxin produces cancer and "serious physiological disorders" in monkeys.

He describes dioxin as the chemical equivalent of plutonium, the most deadly radioactive substance.

An expert on the military history of herbicides, Bruce F. Meyers, a former U.S. Marine colonel, traces their origin to the early years of World War II. At the University of Chicago, what were then categorized as "growth regulators" were seen as being "plant killers." By 1943 the U.S. Army was doing "research in earnest toward the military applications of herbicides in war," notes Meyers.

The outcome was, among other poisons, the development of 2,4-D and 2,4,5-T—numbers and letters which spell death to living things.

"Herbicides were not used in World War II," Meyers continues, but a "program for screening potential herbicides for possible military use continued after the war." And in 1959 "the first large-scale military defoliation by aerial application" using 2,4-D and 2,4,5-T occurred at Fort Drum in upstate New York. "The success of these tests spurred the office of Secretary of Defense Robert McNamara in May of 1961 to request feasibility tests for defoliation of jungle vegetation in Vietnam."

Meanwhile, commercial production of the war-born poisons had begun to boom—with millions of pounds of both toxins being manufactured annually by 1960.

Several mixtures of 2,4-D and 2,4,5-T were sent to Vietnam, and they were code-named by the color of bands painted around the center of the 55-gallon drums in which they were packed. First came Agents Purple and Blue, then Pink and Green, and then Agent Orange which became the primary herbicide used.

Agent Orange, half 2,4-D, half 2,4,5-T, was principally sprayed from huge C-123 aircraft each carrying a thousand gallons of the poison. In "herbicide spraying missions" called Operation Ranch Hand, says Meyers, from 1962 to 1971 some 3.6 million acres of Vietnam were doused with 17.7 million gallons of herbicides.

The spraying program's purpose was "defoliation of trees and plants to improve observation and prevent ambush," he recounts, and to destroy "food crops of hostile forces."

To Michael Ryan, now a police sergeant on Long Island, New York it was "corporate genocide" brought about by institutions which "believed profit is worth more than human life."

"We tried the Germans in Nuremburg. Who is going to try us?" asks the officer.

In 1966, Ryan, 19, was sent with his Army unit to build a camp in a Vietnamese jungle. Aircraft dumping Agent Orange circled nearby as they worked.

Ryan quickly exhibited a sharp weight loss and began feeling the standard effects of Agent Orange which he has been suffering ever since: "excruciating headaches," night sweat, an inability to take even a drop of alcohol, hearing loss. "I don't know how long I'm going to live," Ryan says darkly.

His greatest anxiety is over the daughter born after he returned from Vietnam. Kerry was born with 18 separate genetic defects including double reproductive organs, blindness, no rectum, leakage of blood from the heart, missing fingers.

"I feel hurt, I feel betrayed, I feel very angry," says Ryan.

"The last eight years of my life never had to be," adds his wife, Maureen. "My daughter had the right to be born whole."

Says Maureen Ryan: "The veterans who served their country have been betrayed and are now reaping a harvest of birth defects for their children and cancer for themselves. Society gives business the license to operate but there has been a terrible violation of this public trust." The "astronomically high" chances that Michael Ryan will now develop cancer, the continuing misery for Kerry, the "choice made for us never to have any more children, never to pass on our name" is but "our story" amidst tens of thousands of other Agent Orange horror stories. "The more you get into it, the more the nightmare that comes out."

Most shocking of all to the Ryans has been the arrogance of those responsible: corporations and government.

"I feel like it's another cover-up," Ryan was saying of the denial of fault by the makers of Agent Orange—the largest being Dow Chemical—and the government's collaboration. "I'm a cop and I work with the preponderance of evidence," Ryan says, and the evidence proving the enormous lethality of Agent Orange "is an avalanche."

A class action suit was brought before the U.S. Supreme Court over what happened to the Ryans and other veterans and their families from Agent Orange.

IN THE

Supreme Court of the United States

OCTOBER TERM, 1980

No. 80-1882

◆

CHARLES CHAPMAN, et al.,

Petitioners,

vs.

THE DOW CHEMICAL COMPANY, et al.,

Respondents.

◆

**BRIEF IN SUPPORT OF PETITION
FOR A WRIT OF CERTIORARI
OF THE RYAN FAMILY ON BEHALF OF
ALL THE PLAINTIFF VETERANS AND THEIR
FAMILIES FROM NEW YORK, ALABAMA,
ALASKA, ARKANSAS, COLORADO, GEORGIA,
IDAHO, MAINE, MISSISSIPPI, MONTANA,
NEBRASKA, NEVADA, NORTH CAROLINA,
NORTH DAKOTA, SOUTH DAKOTA, RHODE
ISLAND, UTAH, VIRGINIA, WEST VIRGINIA,
WISCONSIN, AMICI CURIAE**

INTEREST OF AMICI CURIAE

The interest of the *amici curiae* appears from the foregoing motion.

STATEMENT OF THE CASE

This litigation arises out of the use of phenoxy herbicides, including a certain "Agent Orange," which were manufactured, formulated, advertised, marketed, promoted and sold by the multinational, conglomerate, corporate defendant war contractors. The plaintiffs are the class of all those United States veterans who served in Southeast Asia during the "Viet Nam War" and were exposed to chemical defoliants such as the "dioxin" contaminated phenoxy herbicides, together with their wives and children, and, in certain unfortunate cases, their widows, orphans, and parents. See, Appendix B.

The phenoxy herbicides supplied by the defendant War Contractor were admittedly contaminated with polychlorinated dibenzo p-dio (PCDDs), including 2,3,7,8-tetracholoro-dibenzo p-dioxin (TCDD "Dioxin"), a compound conceded to be one of the most toxic substances ever developed by man. See, Appendix C. As a result of exposure to there contaminated herbicides, individual veterans have suffered genetic and somatic damage, including neoplastic disease (cancer). Children of the plaintiff veterans have been born with catastrophic polygenetic birth defects, while others have died *in utero*, been stillborn, or succembed as infants.

In addition to compensatory, general and punitive damages the plaintiff veterans demand declaratory judgment and equitable relief including the creation of a trust fund for the benefit of the afflicted victims out of the current earnings of the corporate defendants rather than out of the public treasury.

Such a trust fund is necessary to assure restitution to, among others, the American taxpayers for benefits paid those victims through the United States Department of Health and Welfare, the social services agencies of the several states and the Veterans Administration. The trust fund may also provide the means for the corporate defendants to avoid economic disaster should the plaintiff veterans and their families ever recover damages consistent with the magnitude of their injuries.

The U.S. government and the corporations involved vigorously fought the lawsuit and on December 15, 1981 the Supreme court rejected it.

A few weeks earlier, Robert Nimmo, administrator of the Veterans Administration, testified before a Senate committee that if the government would compensate Vietnam veterans and their families for the impact of Agent Orange, "We would be looking at hundreds of millions of dollars per year, going into the middle of the next century." Thus, Nimmo told the Senate Veterans Affairs Committee, his agency rejected a proposed government-sponsored study of the effects of Agent Orange.

And the agency continues to refuse to honor the claims of Agent Orange-contaminated vets and their families.

"It is obvious that there is some definite less-than-honorable agreement that has been made between the chemical companies and the bureaucrats," says Yannacone.

Declares W. Keith Kavenagh, also an attorney on the Agent Orange case: "The Nixon administration may have lost the war in Vietnam, but the Reagan administration has won the battle against veterans who came back maimed."

"It is clear that this administration is selling out these young men who answered their country's call to go to Southeast Asia," says Yannacone.

But that is the way it has been all along with Agent Orange from administration to administration.

Agent Orange's corporate manufacturers—Dow and other major chemical companies of America including Hercules, Monsanto, Diamond Shamrock, Uniroyal—steadfastly denied the danger of their product or minimized it, and the government went along. Finally, in 1971 when mounting evidence of the harm Agent Orange was doing became too obvious to ignore, the government halted Agent Orange warfare—too late for the army of its civilian and military victims.

When, in 1976, Maude DeVictor, a counselor at a Veterans Administration hospital in Chicago, made the connection between Vietnam veterans at the facility suffering from types of cancer generally associated with the elderly and their contamination by Agent Orange, the government didn't want to hear about it. Instead, whistle-blower DeVictor was harassed and left government service.

"We each have to take a stand," she maintained. "The chemical companies are killing daily."

And not just with Agent Orange in Southeast Asia.

It is not just the "young men who answered their country's call to go to Southeast Asia" who are the victims.

It is everybody and all life.

For the Agent Orange pattern repeats . . . and repeats.

The Poisoners

They are well-organized, well-financed and they mean business: the poison business.

Take the National Agricultural Chemicals Association. It describes itself as "organized in 1933 to promote the interests of manufacturers and formulators of agricultural chemicals. The primary purpose of the National Agricultural Chemicals Association is to provide a collective industrial force to advance the level of public understanding of the value of pesticides."

Heavily financed by the major chemical companies, it boosts pesticide use through, among other means, what it notes as "a high level of public relations activity"—"public service messages" regularly broadcast on "about 200 U.S. television stations," annual "media tours" which "successfully employ a stable of independent scientific and agricultural spokespeople who visit with media around the country," programs in schools including "a basic course on toxicology for high schools," numerous conferences, a slick feature film "seen in theaters, on television, in schools and in special group showings across the country," and intense lobbying.

Jack D. Early, the president of the National Agricultural Chemicals Association, is constantly on the move—lobbying, promoting, pitching.

During the summer of 1981 he was busy speaking against proposals for the disclosure of company test data about pesticides—what federal and state governments depend on in passing on pesticides, for they do little research of their own. At the most, such information should be "only in a public reading room" where it "could not be copied, reproduced or removed." he told the House Subcommittee on Department Operations, Research and Foreign Agriculture.

```
                          STATEMENT OF
                   DR. JACK D. EARLY, PRESIDENT,
            NATIONAL AGRICULTURAL CHEMICALS ASSOCIATION
                           BEFORE THE
               SUBCOMMITTEE ON DEPARTMENT OPERATIONS,
                   RESEARCH AND FOREIGN AGRICULTURE
                             OF THE
                     COMMITTEE ON AGRICULTURE,
               UNITED STATES HOUSE OF REPRESENTATIVES
                          JUNE 16, 1981
```

Mr. Chairman: I am Jack D. Early, President of the National Agricultural Chemicals Association (NACA). Accompanying me are Mr. Nicholas Reding of Monsanto Company, Chairman of our Board of Directors, and Mr. John D. Conner, our General Counsel.

The member companies of NACA produce virtually all the pesticides used in the United States for agricultural purposes -- both the basic pest control chemicals and the end-use pesticides formulated from these basic chemicals.

NACA is extremely concerned with diminishing property rights in data. We are anxious to see this process reversed by Congress.

As Maureen Hinkle, policy analyst for the National Audubon Society, countered at the same hearing: "The public has a right to know if this residue is going to be in their food and their drinking water. I think they have a right to know what EPA based its decision on and not just to sit with an industry summary in a sealed room."

Early was also protesting against states enacting standards on pesticides stronger than the weak federal regulations.

STATEMENT OF
DR. JACK D. EARLY, PRESIDENT
NATIONAL AGRICULTURAL CHEMICALS ASSOCIATION,
BEFORE THE
SUBCOMMITTEE ON DEPARTMENT OPERATIONS,
RESEARCH AND FOREIGN AGRICULTURE
OF THE
COMMITTEE ON AGRICULTURE,
UNITED STATES HOUSE OF REPRESENTATIVES
JUNE 18, 1981

Mr. Chairman: I am Jack D. Early, President of the National Agricultural Chemicals Association (NACA). Accompanying me are Mr. Nicholas L. Reding, Chairman of our Board of Directors, and Mr. John D. Conner, our General Counsel.

The member companies of NACA produce virtually all the pesticides used in the United States for agricultural purposes -- both the basic pest control chemicals and the end-use pesticides formulated from these basic chemicals.

NACA would like to address Section 24(a) of FIFRA and the compelling need for that authority to be reviewed by this Congress. NACA remains concerned that certain state regulatory activities, and indeed potential trends in this area, have imposed and shall present numerous impediments to the sale and use of pesticide products in the fifty states.

Section 24(a) of the Act, in pertinent part, authorizes states to ". . . regulate the sale or use of any federally registered pesticide . . ." This grant of power has been used by many states to establish far more stringent standards than those required by an agency of the federal government.

Early went on: "It must be emphasized, all pesticide regulations are ultimately paid for at the supermarket check-out register." He did not note that the use of pesticides is ultimately paid for, too, in what the government and industry euphemistically refer to as "health effects."

He declared:

The primary issue to be addressed is the "inherent" authority
of the states to establish data and risk assessment standards that
differ from those established by the federal agency. Some state
assessments are unreasonably based upon vastly expanded research
data submissions -- not only EPA's data, but all research data.

Patricia Wells, staff attorney for the Environmental Defense Fund, replied at that hearing that "states ought to have the right to question EPA's data, to say this is incorrect, it is insufficient, we want more for our people.

"The agricultural chemical industry and its allies cannot be expected to be enthusiastic," she said, about steps to "eliminate the unnecessary use of chemicals and substitute for pesticides other pest control methods which are cheaper, safer, and equally effective. But that is no reason for Congress to put obstacles in the path of a state which wishes to pursue those goals."

Then there is the Chemical Manufacturers Association.
Its literature includes a pamphlet entitled "Food Additives: Who Needs Them?" which includes these pages:

"How can you prove food additives are *absolutely* safe?"

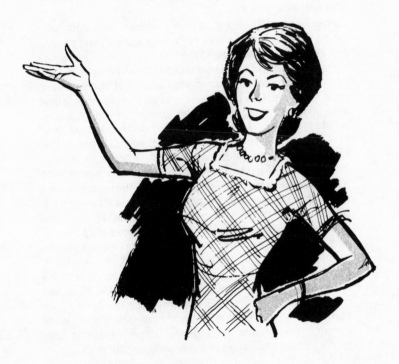

First, what is absolutely safe? Is a safety pin, knife, power motor, auto—or even a horse absolutely safe for the user? And, what about a bicycle, boat or airplane? Or, how 'bout a camp fire . . . or a kitchen range? Yes, the point is simple—it's how one uses a product that determines its safety.

Aristotle said long ago that it is impossible to prove a negative
. . . and safety is a negative. It is the absence of harm. No
matter how many tests one carries out without demonstrating
harm from either a man-made or natural additive, it is always
possible that another test might demonstrate some un-
foreseen harmful effect. For chemical compounds put in food
by man or nature, it's generally how much is ingested which
determines hazard or lack of hazard. Even the so-called
natural, unprocessed foods such as potatoes and cress contain poisons; and cabbage, lettuce, onions, spinach and tea
contain carcinogenic compounds. Yet, these poisons are usually safely digested because they occur at such low levels in
these foods that the human detoxification system functions
appropriately.

Remember that there are no safe or unsafe food additives,
merely safe and unsafe levels of use or ways of using them.
The study of such levels, and the effects of processing, cooking and ingesting chemical compounds put in foods by man or
nature is the work of toxicologists, analytical chemists and
other scientists. This is a never-ending task. Advances in one
area stimulate study and greater learning in others. Some
substances—such as selenium salts—earlier declared toxic
at all levels have since been found not only safe but, below
specific levels, are essential for health. After years of use,
cyclamates were banned as food additives; more reliable tests
may prove these sweeteners entirely safe. The reverse is also
true. Table salt is very toxic above the very low level our taste
buds tolerate. This is why babies—with undeveloped taste
reactions—accept without objection fatal doses of salt in milk
formulas. Consumers often find it confusing when scientific
experts disagree, but this is the way scientific knowledge is
developed. However, it is reassuring to note that due to the
dedication of scientists employed by industry, universities and
government and to the natural detoxification systems of our
bodies, there have been no known or proven occurrences of
cancer, birth deformities, or genetic defects resulting from
food additives consumed in the normal diets of man.

This group would have people believe that even the most
toxic food additives are not "safe or unsafe," it's just how
they are used.

Of foods not doused with chemicals and regarded as "health foods," the Chemical Manufacturers Association insists that an interest in them has to do with "emotions."

"Why such interest in health foods?"

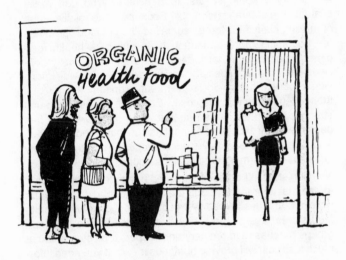

Good question ... the answer's not easy, for it ties in with man's emotions more than with reason. Studying the question is interesting, for man attributed special beliefs and/or powers to foods through the centuries, such as:

- An early "consumer," Nero, ate leeks (onions) seven days each month to clear his voice.

- Lettuce, years ago, was said to clear the senses.

- The tomato was first sold as a decorative plant. In earliest colonial times, it was considered poisonous. But Mediterranean people circulated the idea that the tomato spurred passions.

- In 1632, a London grocer's display of the first banana caused great concern by the pharmacists who maintained the fruit was a deadly drug and to be sold only by trained druggists.

- And in the 1970's a U.S. news magazine reported that a South African headmistress of a girls' high school banned peanut-butter sandwiches "because they were apt to arouse the animal appetites of the young ladies under her charge."

We all have some special food beliefs. Who can really evaluate the above statements? Because of the relative ease of making claims for foods, so-called "health food" products are becoming more abundant. If an attractive health food promoter proclaims that today's foods are nutritionally deficient and his/her "special health foods" will provide more vitality, cure arthritis or increase beauty, consumers often buy them even if they're more costly. Emotions are usually much stronger than reason. It's true that some of this emotion has been fueled by excessive or inept use of some food additives. And some of these have quite properly had their safety questioned—as must continually be done.

Nutritionists don't object if so-called health foods are bought for their taste or texture. But, they are disturbed if consumers believe that a healthy family diet can be bought only in health food stores. It is still true that diets based on the four food groups purchased in ordinary and "super" food stores and at much less cost will provide nutritious meals. If you need information to plan better meals, consult your county extension home economist, Food and Drug Administration consumer affairs officer or a home economics teacher.

As to "the amount of additives used?" Five pounds *spread over a year, is that huge?* (Spread over a lifetime, 300 to 400 pounds of additives might not sound that huge either—or does it?)

"How 'bout a few words on the amount of additives used?"

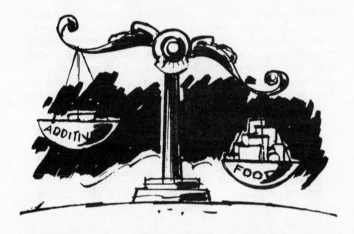

1) *What about the huge amount of additives that we consume?* Let's first look at that word "huge." Our per capita consumption of food in 1970 was 1,500 pounds of which five pounds were additives of all kinds. Spread over a year, is that huge? And, remember, "natural—no additives" doesn't mean no chemicals. Natural grape flavor, for example, contains at least 19 identified chemical compounds, as compared with only five of the major components of these in the synthetic version.

2) *Yes, but what about the pounds of synthetic food colors that are used every year in dairy products, beverages, baked goods, spices, jellies, candy, cereals, meat-product casings, maraschino cherries and even Easter egg dyes?* According to the National Academy of Sciences/National Research Council, the total consumption of these is only about 0.012 pounds (5.5 grams) per person every year. In addition to chronic studies already performed, producers have conducted thorough teratolog-

ical and multigeneration studies on all of the certified food colors. To date, these tests have shown no adverse effects. However, all color additives are subject to constant scrutiny and retesting by both industry and the Food and Drug Administration. Should any doubt arise regarding the safety of a color additive, such color is immediately removed from the list of regulated additives until the question of its safety can be resolved by competent scientific authorities.

NOTE: Some unfavorable effects have been observed in animals fed BHA and BHT in substantial amounts—1,000 to 5,000 parts per million in the total diet. However, scientists estimate that using BHT or BHA at the prescribed maximum level in *all* foods in which authorized would yield a maximum daily intake of about four parts per million (ppm)—an entirely safe level. Actual usage is substantially less. These studies consider cumulative effects in the test animals and the human detoxification system.

Separately, the huge chemical companies themselves get into the act. Monsanto has a booklet aiming to assure people about toxic chemicals products by insisting "life is risky" anyway.

Chemical Risk: The Other Half of the Story

Life is risky. When our cavemen stoked their first fire, they risked burns. Modern life has reduced some risks but increased others.

A risk is the possibility of loss or injury. Every one of us continually makes decisions which involve risks.

Every time a person climbs stairs, mows a lawn, handles a pet, plays a sport, crosses a street or rides in a car, there is risk. These situations, where the risk of harm is immediate, are called acute risks. Other risks are not so obvious or immediate. They are called chronic risks. Exposure to noise over a long time increases the chances of impaired hearing — a chronic risk.

Do chemicals cause risks? Obviously some do. Many chemicals are highly poisonous. Others can explode violently. Both of those examples are acute chemical risks. Evidence indicates that exposure to some chemicals over a long period increases the chance of illness. So there are chronic risks, too.

The chemical industry generally has done a good job recognizing acute risks and taking the necessary steps to protect employees and the public. The safety record in chemical plants is among the best in all industry.

Monsanto's slogan is "without chemicals, life itself is impossible." The other half of that is *with* the poisonous chemicals that Monsanto and the other giant chemical corporations are peddling, life for many people has become impossible.

Then there is the poison press, from *Food Chemical News...*

FOOD CHEMICAL NEWS

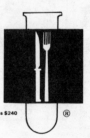

A weekly Washington publication for executives providing in-depth information regarding regulation of food additives, colors, pesticides, and allied products.

$390 a year Additional subscriptions $240 ®

Volume 23, Number 38 ● November 30, 1981

HIGHLIGHTS of the news

SODIUM dual declaration on food labels to be eliminated by FDA.	Page 25
EEC MEAT INSPECTION requirements eased in revised draft.	Page 26
IRRADIATION emergency Medfly use FDA final approval withheld.	Page 22
CRANBERRY JUICE DRINK labeling pressure applied to FDA.	Page 33

to *Farm Chemicals . . .*

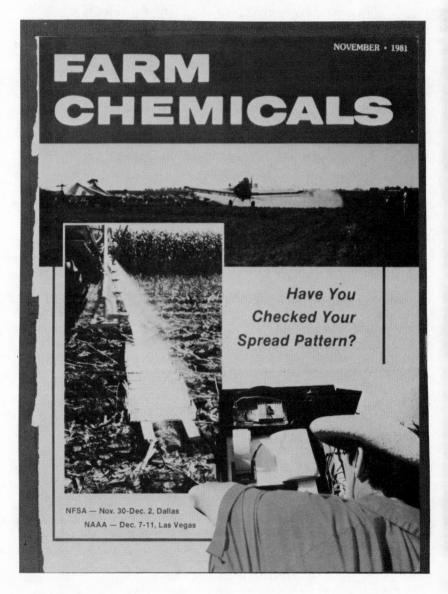

. . . chock full of these kinds of ads:

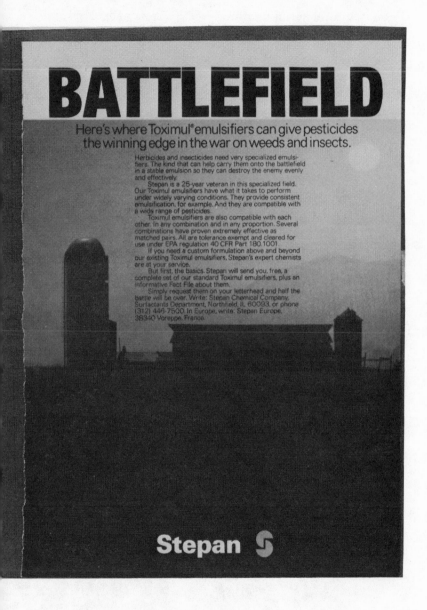

BATTLEFIELD

Here's where Toximul® emulsifiers can give pesticides the winning edge in the war on weeds and insects.

Herbicides and insecticides need very specialized emulsifiers. The kind that can help carry them onto the battlefield in a stable emulsion so they can destroy the enemy evenly and effectively.

Stepan is a 25-year veteran in this specialized field. Our Toximul emulsifiers have what it takes to perform under widely varying conditions. They provide consistent emulsification, for example. And they are compatible with a wide range of pesticides.

Toximul emulsifiers are also compatible with each other. In any combination and in any proportion. Several combinations have proven extremely effective as matched pairs. All are tolerance exempt and cleared for use under EPA regulation 40 CFR Part 180.1001.

If you need a custom formulation above and beyond our existing Toximul emulsifiers, Stepan's expert chemists are at your service.

But first, the basics. Stepan will send you, free, a complete set of our standard Toximul emulsifiers, plus an informative Fact File about them.

Simply request them on your letterhead and half the battle will be over. Write: Stepan Chemical Company, Surfactants Department, Northfield, IL 60093, or phone (312) 446-7500. In Europe, write: Stepan Europe, 38340 Voreppe, France.

Stepan 🌀

A chemical company's view of the balance of nature.

Agricultural aerial warfare.

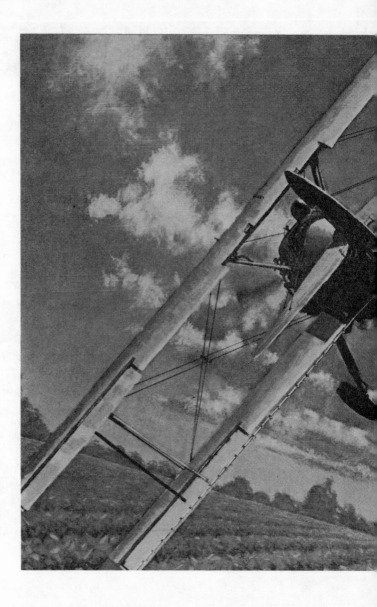

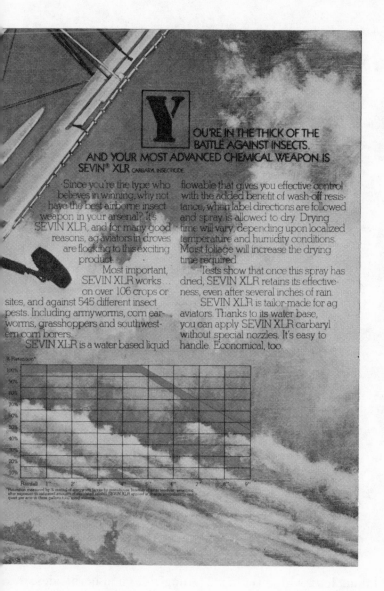

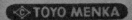
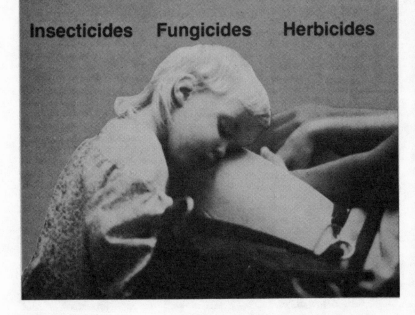
Linking love with insecticides, fungicides and herbicides.

The editor of *Farm Chemicals,* Gordon L. Berg, regularly rails against suggestions that anything might be wrong with chemical farming.

In the September 1981 issue, Berg hit at The Cornucopia Project sponsored by the Rodale Press, publisher of *Organic Gardening.* The Cornucopia Project's aims are to provide information to lower food costs and to help facilitate organic agriculture. What the project involves would mean a return to the "glory days of the past," complained Berg, "organic farming no less." It is "inconceivable to us," he protested, that the Rodale project receives so much attention." He noted the comment of the "outstanding agricultural researcher," Dr. Keith Huston, at an Association of State Agricultural Experiment Station Directors gathering—sponsored by the Velsicol Chemical Corp.—that "we're living in the age of science and if you're not in step with it, you're hopelessly out of touch."

And there's *Food Technology,* published by the Institute of Food Technologists which describes itself as a 19,500-member "educational and scientific society of food professionals—technologists, scientists, engineers, educators and executives—in the field of food technology."

From the pages of *Food Technology:*

Eat your heart out Mother Nature, indeed.

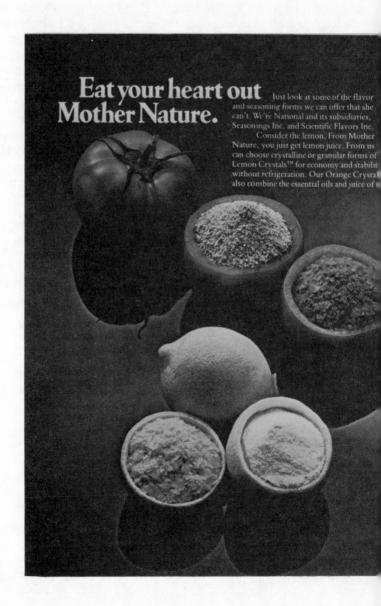

Eat your heart out Mother Nature.

Just look at some of the flavor and seasoning forms we can offer that she can't. We're National and its subsidiaries, Seasonings Inc. and Scientific Flavors Inc.

Consider the lemon. From Mother Nature, you just get lemon juice. From us can choose crystalline or granular forms of Lemon Crystals™ for economy and stabilit without refrigeration. Our Orange Crystal also combine the essential oils and juice of

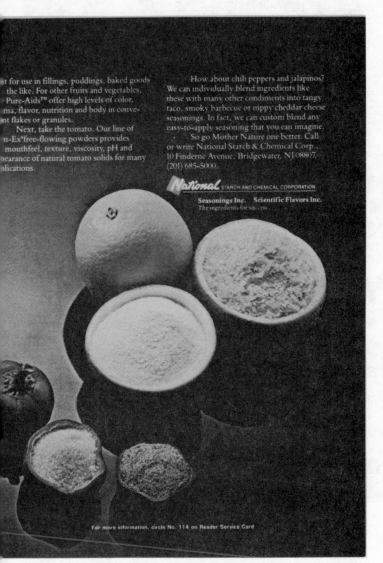

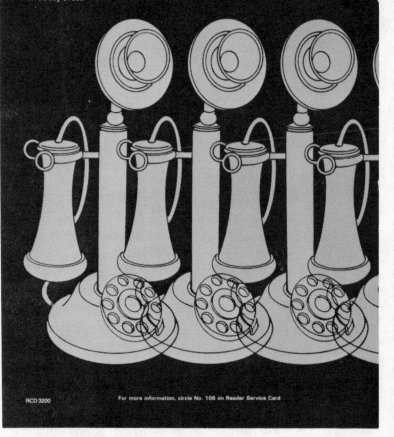
Touch tone toxins?

CHOCOLIM II

A new artificial chocolate flavor — Chocolim II is offered for use in ice cream, yogurt, beverages, candies, and all other foods in which natural chocolate is generally used. This liquid chocolate flavor can be used as a partial or total replacement for natural chocolate flavor which has been constantly rising in price. A low rate of usage is required for this product, ie. ½ ounce to make 1 gallon of ice cream mix; in beverages 3 ounces to 1 gallon of syrup, 1 to 2 ounces per 100 lbs of artificial chocolate coatings, etc.

Artificial Chocolate Oil

One ounce of this synthetic oil can replace about seven lbs of cocoa at a considerable saving in cost.

BRANCHES WORLDWIDE

RITTER INTERNATIONAL

GENERAL OFFICES AND MANUFACTURING:
4001-09 GOODWIN AVENUE/LOS ANGELES, CALIFORNIA 90039/USA/AREA CODE 213-245-6886

Better chocolate through chemistry?

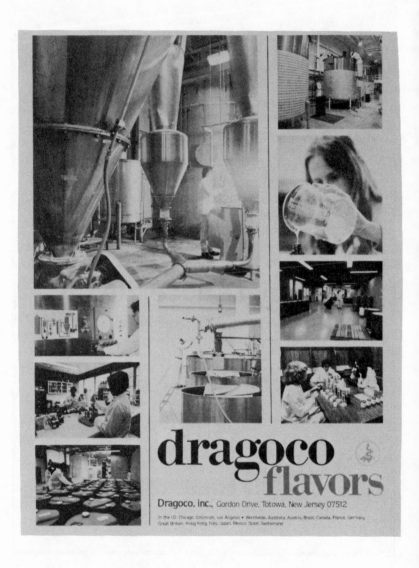

Food fresh from the laboratory.

In editorials in *Food Technology*, Arthur T. Schramm, president of The Institute of Food Technologists, defends chemicalized food. In the December 1981 issue writing on "The Food Safety Debate," Schramm noted that there have been "doubts about the safety of our food supply" in recent years and "particular attention has been directed to specific food additives and environmental contamination.

"When we read about the 'carcinogen of the month' in our food supply, we sense a subtle, lurking threat to our health," he noted, but "risks are inherently a part of life" and "we must learn to cope with uncertainties, since decisions concerning socially acceptable risk must be made for ingredients in our food supply, whether they are normal components, additives, environmental contaminants, natural toxicants, pesticides, or packaging constituents which transfer to food. Such decisions are social and political in nature and must be made on the basis of limited and uncertain scientific information."

The Institute of Food Technologists puts out other material including a pamphlet entitled "Quick Answers to Commonly Asked Questions about Food." Some excerpts:

Are artificial colors and flavors bad for you?

No. Each one in commercial use has been accepted as safe by the U.S. Food & Drug Administration. In the quantities used, none has ever been demonstrated to cause harm. There simply are not enough of either natural colors or natural flavors available to produce the quantity and variety of foods which American consumers demand. Artificial colors and flavors help fill this demand.

What foods are suspected of causing cancer?

No foods are really "suspected of causing cancer," although charges have been leveled against certain food additives, based on isolated tests bearing little or no resemblance to eating habits. These include nitrites in cured meats (after they presumably react with other chemicals in the gut), certain food colors, and synthetic sweeteners. The same charges could be aimed at many natural foods: sassafras contains safrol; leafy vegetables contain nitrate; shrimp even contain arsenic. At the levels we actually eat, none of these products, natural or synthetic, have ever been shown to cause cancer.

. . . none of these products . . . have ever been shown to cause cancer, claims the Institute of Food Technologists.

As in the case of Agent Orange—it is deny, deny, deny.

The chemical industry is also deeply involved in the funding of what is supposed to look like a consumers group, the American Council on Science and Health.

Its guru is Dr. Frederick Stare, who through huge grants and gifts from food companies such as Borden, Kellogg and General Foods brought a nutrition department he started at the Harvard School of Public Health into prominence and went on to compensate his benefactors by defending U.S. food practices, particularly the extensive use of sugar in processed foods.

A former student and employee, Elizabeth Murphy Whelan, is the group's executive director. Stare is on the board.

Explains Peter Harnick of a real consumers group, the Center for Science in the Public Interest in Washington, the Whelan-Stare operation will choose "a pesticide such as 2,4,5-T or a food additive such as caffeine that is being criticized as a health hazard" and will come up with a report claiming "the substance is safe—or rather that there is no evidence to show that it isn't safe—if used in a reasonable manner by a reasonable person; issues a flurry of press releases ballyhooing the finding; criticizes regulatory agencies for considering restricting the substance" and then "parlays its position into additional financial support" from its corporate benefactors.

"We're not paid off to say anything," Mrs. Whelan contends. "We don't feel a chemical is guilty until proven innocent" and "we don't think a chemical should be banned at the drop of a rat." She set up the group in Washington in 1978.

In a speech at Hillsdale College in Michigan in 1980, she maintained that "today's consumer advocates" were leading the way to "not only zero risk, but zero food, zero jobs, zero energy and zero growth" and said that "for executives in the chemical industry, the burden falls particularly hard" but "some companies, like Monsanto and General Foods, have already taken the initiative" with "public education."

The Whelan-Stare group "with its $750,000 budget espouses positions nearly identical to those of its corporate sponsors," notes Harnick.

Michael Jacobson, executive director of the Center for Science in the Public Interest describes the Whelan-Stare organization as "a front for industry."

The poisoners leave no stone unturned to climb under as they push their toxins.

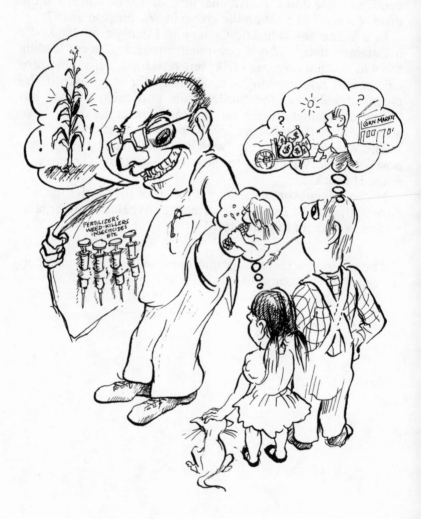

Admitted Consequences

The admitted consequences from the toxins being wantonly spread through our environment have been growing—although still what is being conceded is the tip of a poisonous iceberg of global reach.

Cancer is the No. 1 admitted effect of the monkey wrench of poison being thrown into nature's cycle.

As this 1980 report of a Presidential Toxic Substances Strategy Committee concluded, *environmental factors . . . are significant in the great majority of cancer cases seen, perhaps 80–90 percent.*

It declared:

> Of the hazards to human health arising from toxic substances, cancer is a leading source of concern. Cancer is the only major cause of death that has continued to rise since 1900. It is now second only to heart disease as a cause of death and is responsible for the loss of 400,000 lives each year. Some of the increase in cancer mortality since 1900 is a function of the greater average age of the U.S. population and the medical progress made against infectious disease. But even after correcting for age, both mortality (death) rates and incidence (new cases) of cancer are increasing.
>
> Many now believe that environmental (nongenetic) factors—life style and work and environmental exposures—are significant in the great majority of cancer cases seen, perhaps 80–90 percent. Cancers appear to be multi-staged, and various environmental factors may affect different stages in the progression to malignancy.

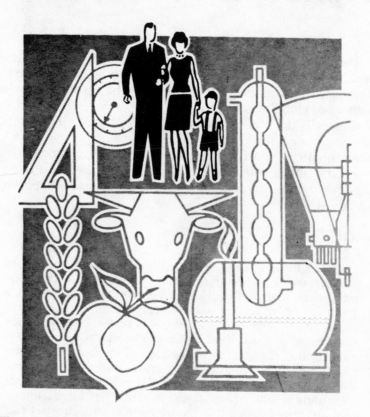

May 1980

Toxic Chemicals and Public Protection

A Report to
the President
by the
Toxic
Substances
Strategy
Committee

The report went on:

Human exposure to toxic substances may occur through air, water, and terrestrial pollution; through pesticides, foods and food additives, drugs, cosmetics, consumer products, workplace conditions, waste disposal, and accidents. Perhaps the most serious source of human exposure to toxic chemicals is the workplace. Many workers die each year as a result of physical and chemical hazards at work, but the exact magnitude of the long-term health effects of occupational conditions is unknown. Occupational exposure to carcinogens is believed to be a factor in more than 20 percent of all cases of cancer. An unknown number of persons is at risk because of hazardous chemicals seeping into water supplies from hazardous waste dump sites across the nation and because of many other types of exposure.

And in addition to cancer:

Human health effects include cancer, birth defects and other reproductive anomalies, neurological and behavioral disorders, kidney damage, lung and heart disease, acute and chronic skin disease, and acute poisoning. Certain subtle effects, such as on intelligence, may be totally undetected. For example, the immediate effects of high level exposures for a short time include burns, rashes, nausea, loss of eyesight, and fatal poisoning. Prolonged exposure to low doses can cause chronic lung disease (e.g., from coal or cotton dust), heart disease (from exposure to cadmium or carbon monoxide), sterility (from dibromochloropropane—DBCP), and kidney, liver, brain, nerve, or other damage. Exposure to industrial solvents can cause depression, and carbon disulfide is associated with a higher suicide rate among workers than in the general population. Although most chemicals do not cause cancer, exposure to some has been linked to cancer. Some workers exposed to asbestos, even for a short time, have developed a rare cancer of the chest and stomach linings 30–40 years after initial exposure. Vinyl chloride gas is linked to a rare liver cancer, to a brain cancer, and possibly to lung cancer. Diethylstilbestrol (DES), when taken by pregnant women to prevent miscarriage, led to increased risk of vaginal cancer in their daughters and abnormal sexual organs in their sons. Methyl mercury, formed by the action of bacteria in sediments on mercury metal and on mercuric ions, can cause acute poisoning, deafness, brain damage, and a range of birth defects. A single substance can have several kinds of adverse effects, depending on the route and level of exposure.

This report included a graph of what pollutants are generally connected to what diseases:

FIRST ANNUAL REPORT TO CONGRESS

BY

**THE TASK FORCE ON
ENVIRONMENTAL CANCER AND HEART AND LUNG DISEASE**

ENVIRONMENTAL POLLUTION
AND
CANCER AND HEART AND LUNG DISEASE

Washington, D.C.
August 7, 1978

U. S. Environmental Protection Agency
National Cancer Institute
National Heart, Lung and Blood Institute
National Institute for Occupational Safety & Health
National Institute of Environmental Health Sciences

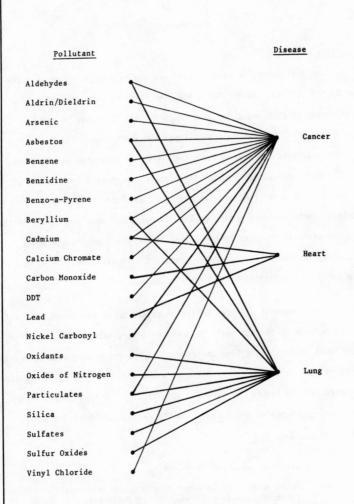

Figure 2. Known or Suspected Links Between Selected Pollutants and Disease

Said this study: *The environment we have created may now be a major cause of death in the United States.*

THE PROBLEM

INTRODUCTION

The environment we have created may now be a major cause of death in the United States. Cancer, heart and lung disease, accounting for 12 percent of deaths in 1900 and 38 percent in 1940, were the cause of 59 percent of all deaths in 1976. Patterns of illness and death have changed over the years. Medical advances have reduced the impact of infection and accident, and life expectancy has increased. After other causes of illness and death have been brought under control, cancer, heart and lung disease have emerged as dominant factors in the public health. Growing evidence links much of the occurrence of these diseases to the nature of the environment. National levels of illness might be sharply reduced, and life prolonged, if we could better manage our relations with the environment.

Environmental chemical pollution refers to compounds which impact upon the human body through their occurrence in air, water, soil, or other media. This definition implies the possibility of preventing adverse health effects of pollutant exposure by measures which eliminate the pollutant from the environment or reduce its impact. Specifically for this year's report, the following categories are included in the definition of environmental chemical pollution:

- Airborne gases and particulates

- Toxic substances in water supplies and in contact surfaces such as clothing, foliage, and paint.

- Pesticides and herbicides

- Chemical contaminants in food

- Occupational exposures to hazardous substances

- Passive smoking (i.e., in exposure of nonsmokers to smoking of others).

Of the upwards of 100,000 known chemicals of potential toxicity, only approximately 6,000 have been laboratory tested for carcinogenicity. It is estimated that 10 to 16 percent of the chemicals so tested provide some evidence of animal carcinogenicity. To scratch the surface of the complexity which researchers and regulators are faced with, a few inherent problems in cancer research are listed below:

- Cancer in man usually has multifactorial causes.

- The long latent period of cancer has troublesome medical, social and economic implications. Chemicals may appear to be safe for human exposure after being used for 10 to 15 years; this gives a false sense of security.

- Mobility of society poses another problem -- collection of data for epidemiology studies is difficult.

- Tests on animals are expensive and time consuming, and extrapolation of animal data to effects in man is difficult.

- Concentrations of single chemicals in the environment are often low, requiring sensitive methods for detection and analysis.

The *long latent period of cancer* that the investigation cited is crucial: *Chemicals may appear to be safe for human exposure after being used for 10 to 15 years; this gives a false sense of security.*
The dollar costs of environmental disease are immense, the report stressed.

THE COSTS OF ENVIRONMENTAL DISEASE

A recent estimate, 1972, places an approximate value for the total annual costs of cancer, heart and lung disease at about 69 billion dollars annually (Figure 3). These estimates comprise costs of treatment and the value of lost earnings from illness and early death. If even a relatively small percentage of this amount could be saved through reduction of the environmentally related components of these three diseases, the savings to the American public would be immense. The present cost of these diseases, in medical expense and taxes, is a burden which is unacceptable and at least partly avoidable.

The cost savings which might result from an effective solution of
environmentally related disease problems must be considered in conjunction
with the other costs, and social and economic dislocations, which must be
incurred if the levels of pollution in our environment are to be reduced.
The costs of eliminating some pollutants, through industrial source controls
or changing of industrial materials usages, may be small in comparison with
potential benefits in health and health cost savings.

And it included this chart of those costs:

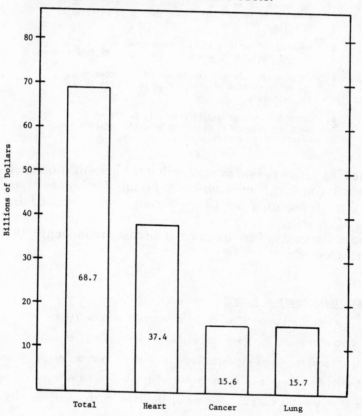

Figure 3. Estimated Health Care Costs for Heart, Cancer and Lung Diseases, 1972 *

And those *tens of billions* of dollars in cost for environmental diseases are based on 1972 dollars—they would be double now!

As the report concluded:

The problem facing the Nation today in regard to environmental cancer, heart and lung disease can be summarized as follows:

- There is evidence that risk and occurrence of cancer, heart and lung disease increase with environmental pollution, broadly defined to include all environmental factors.

- The extent of illness, death, and costs to society from environmentally related cancer, heart and lung disease is a matter of national concern.

- There is expectation that levels of illness, death, and cost resulting from these environmentally related diseases could be substantially reduced by preventive measures.

- Current preventive measures are believed to be inadequate to obtain desired reductions of risk and occurrence.

- Increased knowledge of pollution-disease relations and improvements in strategies and preventive measures are needed for reduction of risk and occurrence.

- The Federal Government has a central, critical role to take in research and prevention of environmentally related diseases; changes in current Federal efforts may be necessary if desired reductions of risk and occurrence of environmentally related cancer, heart and lung disease are to be obtained.

Another document on the consequences of poisons in the environment is this 1979 report of the U.S. Congress's Office of Technology Assessment:

Environmental Contaminants in Food

Summary

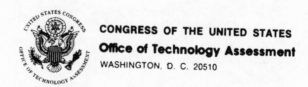

CONGRESS OF THE UNITED STATES
Office of Technology Assessment
WASHINGTON, D. C. 20510

Said the report:

The environmental contamination of food is a nationwide problem. A number of recent incidents dramatically illustrate the potential health hazards and economic harm that can be caused by such contamination—animal feeds in Michigan contaminated by polybrominated biphenyls (PBBs), the Hudson River contaminated by polychlorinated biphenyls (PCBs), and Virginia's James River contaminated by kepone.

These are some of the more serious of the 243 food contamination incidents identified in an OTA survey of the 50 States and 10 Federal agencies. These incidents have occurred in every region of the country. They have involved all categories of food. While the OTA survey clearly shows the national character of such contamination, the true extent of the problem is still unknown.

The latest major food contamination incident—one not included in the OTA survey—graphically points up the national dimensions of the problem. PCBs from a damaged transformer contaminated animal fats at a packing plant in Billings, Mont. The plant used the adulterated fats to produce meat and bone meal that were sold both to feed manufacturers and directly to farmers. The contaminated feed spread through at least 10 States—polluting poultry, eggs, pork products, and a variety of processed foods (including strawberry cake). The result: contaminated food found in 17 States, and hundreds of thousands of pounds of food products seized or destroyed.

As to health consequences:

HEALTH IMPACTS OF ENVIRONMENTAL CONTAMINATION

Four factors determine whether and how seriously the environmental contamination of food will affect human health: the toxicity of the contaminant, the amount of the substance in the food, the amount of the contaminated food eaten, and the physiological vulnerability of the individual or individuals consuming the food.

Based on other countries' experiences, there is considerable evidence of human illness caused by the consumption of food containing various organic chemicals and metals. In such cases, the level of the contaminant in food exceeded the levels usually found in the U.S. food supply. The effects of mercury poisoning are well-documented. The best known case involved the consumption of mercury-contaminated fish from Japan's Minamata Bay. Some of the offspring of exposed mothers were born with birth defects, and many victims suffered central nervous system damage.

Another incident in Japan stemmed from the inadvertent contamination of rice oil by PCBs. The consumption of food cooked with this oil resulted in 1,291 cases of so-called "Yusho disease"—a condition marked by chloracne (a severe form of acne), eye discharges, skin discoloration, headaches, fatigue, abdominal pains, and liver and menstrual disturbances.

No such mass-poisoning episodes have occurred in the United States. But there are studies indicating that present levels of some environmental contaminants may cause physiological changes. For example, the accidental contamination of animal feed in 1973 exposed most of the population of Michigan to PBB in dairy products and other foods.

Our regulatory monitory system has failed to detect such environmental contaminants as they entered the food supply.

To determine whether an environmental contamination incident has occurred, it is necessary to establish the presence of the contaminant in food. In some instances, people or animals have become ill before the responsible contaminant was identified. No one knew or even suspected that the particular substance was present in food. This has been the pattern in many major contamination incidents—those involving PBBs, PCBs, and mercury.

Our regulatory monitoring system has failed to detect such environmental contaminants as they entered the food supply. Thus, this assessment identifies and evaluates other approaches for monitoring either food or the environment for toxic substances that may harm human health. The ultimate objective of monitoring is to prevent or minimize human exposure to environmental contaminants in food.

The only sure way to prevent this kind of contamination is to make certain that toxic substances are not released into the environment. There are various Federal environmental laws that are designed to limit such releases. But the laws and regulations are not likely to prevent the deliberate or accidental misuse or disposal of the thousands of toxic substances manufactured in the United States.

The problem is compounded by disposal and handling practices that were accepted in the past but are now recognized as posing serious environmental hazards—hazards that will persist for many years to come. The toxic chemical waste dump at the Love Canal near Niagara Falls, N. Y., clearly illustrates the threat. According to Environmental Protection Agency (EPA) estimates, there are 1,200 to 2,000 of these abandoned chemical and radioactive waste sites in the United States that pose an imminent danger to human health and will cost as much as $50 billion to clean up. As long as these substances remain in the environment, the potential for food contamination exists.

The only sure way to prevent this kind of contamination is to make certain that toxic substances are not released into the environment.

Declared the U.S. Surgeon General in 1980, the poisoning of America by toxic chemicals is clearly *a major and growing public health problem.*

HEALTH EFFECTS OF TOXIC POLLUTION:
A REPORT FROM THE SURGEON GENERAL

AND

A BRIEF REVIEW OF SELECTED ENVIRONMENTAL
CONTAMINATION INCIDENTS WITH A POTENTIAL
FOR HEALTH EFFECTS

REPORTS

PREPARED BY THE

SURGEON GENERAL
DEPARTMENT OF HEALTH AND HUMAN SERVICES

AND THE

CONGRESSIONAL RESEARCH SERVICE
OF THE
LIBRARY OF CONGRESS

FOR THE

COMMITTEE ON ENVIRONMENT AND
PUBLIC WORKS
U.S. SENATE

AT THE REQUEST OF

SENATOR EDMUND S. MUSKIE
SENATOR JOHN C. CULVER
AND
SENATOR ROBERT T. STAFFORD

AUGUST 1980

A Report from the Department of Health and Human Services
Public Health Service

to the

United States Senate
Committee on Environment and Public Works
Subcommittee on Environmental Pollution

on

ASSESSMENT OF THE THREAT TO PUBLIC HEALTH POSED BY TOXIC CHEMICALS
IN THE UNITED STATES

Background

On April 25, 1980, the Senate Committee on Environment and Public
Works, Subcommittee on Environmental Pollution, asked the Department of
Health and Human Services (DHHS) to respond to the following questions:

o   What efforts has the DHHS undertaken to assess the danger
     to public health posed by toxic chemicals?

o   What is the judgment of the Surgeon General as to the
     extent of the toxics problem as it affects health
     generally, as well as its potential for creating
     public health emergencies?

o   In the opinion of the Surgeon General, is the magnitude
     of the public health risk increasing or decreasing?

While at this time it is impossible to determine the magnitude of
the toxic chemical risk, it is clear that it is a major and growing
public health problem. Efforts to define the magnitude of the problem
more precisely are hampered by two factors: first, the long latent
period that frequently exists between chemical exposure and chemically
induced disease and, second, the newness of the science of environmental
toxicology. Thus, as the problems of toxic chemical waste dumps and
aquifer contamination have shown us, we are currently in the very early
stages of a health problem which may take years to assess fully.

Conclusion

In summary, we believe that toxic chemicals are adding to the
disease burden of the United States in a significant, although as yet
not precisely defined, way. In addition, we believe that this problem
will become more important in the years ahead.

It is our hope and belief that full implementation of recent environmental control legislation will sharply reduce the marketing of toxic
chemicals and consequently reduce the exposure of our people to such

chemicals. However, through this decade we believe we will confront a
series of environmental emergencies.

We believe that the magnitude of the public health risk associated
with toxic chemicals currently is increasing and will continue to do so
until we are successful in identifying chemicals which are highly toxic
and controlling the introduction of these chemicals into our environment.

*We believe that the magnitude of the public health risk
associated with toxic chemicals currently is increasing and
will continue to do so . . .*

Why the Supposed Protectors Don't Protect

"I aimed at the public's heart and by accident I hit it in the stomach," Upton Sinclair wrote after his turn-of-the-century book, *The Jungle,* was an important factor in leading the U.S. government to take its first steps to deal with poison in food. *The Jungle* concerned the filth that accompanied meat production in America and played a large part in causing Congress to pass the Pure Food and Drugs Act and Meat Inspections Act, both in 1906.

In addition to the writings of muckraker Sinclair, the illnesses and deaths among U.S. soldiers who had eaten what was revealed to have been contaminated meat during the Spanish-American War amplified the issue.

And there was the work of Dr. Harvey Washington Wiley, a physician who as chief chemist of the U.S. Department of Agriculture had been charging for years that Americans were being poisoned by dangerous chemicals being added to food.

Also active in pushing for pure food legislation were an early consumer group, the National Consumer League; farmers who comprised a key segment of the Populist movement of the time; George T. Angel, a lawyer otherwise known for attempts to prevent cruelty to animals; the General Federation of Women's Clubs; and other muckraking journalists besides Sinclair.

The nation had undergone a transition from a rural land to an increasingly industrial society in which businesses were being developed to market processed food, usually doused with chemicals.

"Chemicals could be used to heighten color, modify flavor, soften texture, deter spoilage, and even transform ingredients like apple scraps, glucose, coal-tar dye, and timothy seeds into a concoction labeled strawberry jam," relates James Henry Young, an Emory University history processor and a specialist on the period's pure food movement. "Adulteration might be an age-old problem but, in the words of a Senate report in 1890," notes Young, "'it has only been since the great opportunity for fraud provided by modern science . . . that the sophistication of articles of commerce has reached its present height.'"

"By a sort of Gresham's law," says Young, "adulterated foods that could be sold more cheaply threatened to drive out sounder fare."

Young regards Wiley as "the leader of the pure food crusade." Arriving in Washington in 1883, he "made the study of food adulteration his bureau's principal business." Wiley was "at first outraged by what he deemed essentially harmless fraud" but "in time, sensing real threats to health, Wiley could express himself in writing, conversation, and oratory with vividness, clarity, homely wit, and moral passion. He toured the country making speeches, every rostrum a pulpit for the gospel of pure food . . . He sought to organize his allies and recruits into a coalition which might be powerful enough to move Congress to action."

He formed what became known as "Dr. Wiley's Poison Squad," a dozen Department of Agriculture employees who served as volunteer guinea pigs eating doses of commonly-used additives to determine their effects, and stir the public up about the need for a pure food law.

Finally, on June 30, 1906, President Theodore Roosevelt signed the Pure Food and Drugs Act which defined as adulterated foods those containing "any added poisonous or other added deleterious ingredient which may render such article injurious to health."

And Dr. Wiley, who the U.S. government honored in 1956 by issuing a postage stamp with his likeness and who government literature likes to describe as the "father of food and drug regulation," began trying to enforce the law as head of the Bureau of Chemistry of the Department of Agriculture, the forebearer of the Food and Drug Administration.

Fifty-ninth Congress of the United States of America;

At the First Session,

Begun and held at the City of Washington on Monday, the fourth day of December, one thousand nine hundred and five.

AN ACT

For preventing the manufacture, sale, or transportation of adulterated or misbranded or poisonous or deleterious foods, drugs, medicines, and liquors, and for regulating traffic therein, and for other purposes.

Be it enacted by the Senate and House of Representatives of the United States of America in Congress assembled, That it shall be unlawful for any person to manufacture within any Territory or the District of Columbia any article of food or drug which is adulterated or misbranded, within the meaning of this Act; and any person who shall violate any of the provisions of this section shall be guilty of a misdemeanor, and for each offense shall, upon conviction thereof, be fined not to exceed five hundred dollars or shall be sentenced to one year's imprisonment, or both such fine and imprisonment, in the discretion of the court, and for each subsequent offense and conviction thereof shall be fined not less than one thousand dollars or sentenced to one year's imprisonment, or both such fine and imprisonment, in the discretion of the court.

SEC. 2. That the introduction into any State or Territory or the District of Columbia from any other State or Territory or the District of Columbia, or from any foreign country, or shipment to any foreign country of any article of food or drugs which is adulterated or misbranded, within the meaning of this Act, is hereby prohibited; and any person who shall ship or deliver for shipment from any State or Territory or the District of Columbia to any other State or Territory or the District of Columbia, or to a foreign country, or who shall receive in any State or Territory or the District of Columbia from any other State or Territory or the District of Columbia, or foreign country, and having so received, shall deliver, in original unbroken packages, for pay or otherwise,

Intent and political reality became two different things.

Government inspectors, for example, had not been empowered to enter a food processing plant—unless allowed by the plant's management. Penalties were light. Pesticides had come into use containing such poisons as arsenic, but the act didn't cover their incorporation in food and attempts to deal with pesticides were beaten back by industry lobbying.

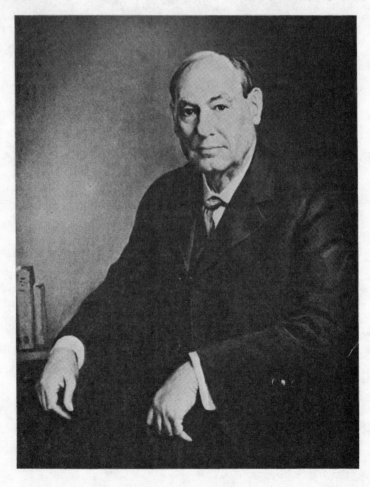

Dr. Harvey W. Wiley

In 1912, as a matter of conscience, Dr. Wiley—after 29 years of government service—resigned. He decided he would be able to more effectively fight against poison in food outside of government.

As he later wrote in his autobiography, *The History of a*

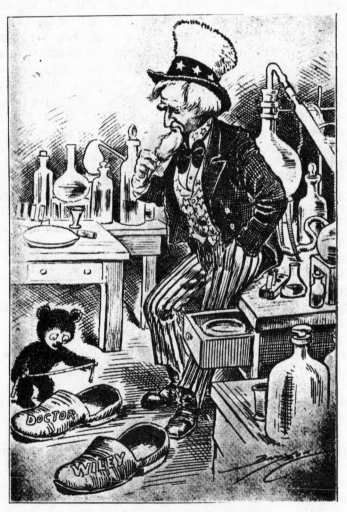

Washington Star cartoon on Dr.
Wiley's resignation

Crime Against the Food Law, the law that was intended to protect the health of the people was "perverted to protect adulteration of food and drugs."

He declared: "There is a distinct tendency to put regulations and rules for the enforcement of the law into the hands of industries engaged in food and drug activities. I consider this one of the most pernicious threats to pure food and drugs. Business is making rapid strides in the control of all our affairs. When we permit business in general to regulate the quality and character of our food and drug supplies, we are treading upon very dangerous ground. It is always advisable to consult business men and take such advice as they give that is unbiased, because of the intimate knowledge they have of the processes involved. It is never advisable to surrender entirely food and drug control to business interests."

During the New Deal, President Franklin D. Roosevelt backed reforms in the Pure Food and Drugs Act and, for five years, battled intense industry pressure until the Food, Drug and Cosmetic Act of 1938 was passed. It stands today, with amendments, as the basic law intended to provide pure food in America. But it, like the 1906 legislation, also turned out to be flawed.

This law, for instance, provided exemptions for poisons added to food if the toxins were deemed "unavoidable" or "necessary in production." There was nothing to require proof that what was put in food was safe.

And so by the late 1940's, with many thousands of new chemicals being added to food, a Congressional inquiry was begun. The World War II explosion in chemical warfare research which led to chemical pesticides had a counterpart in the development for the military of foods heavily treated with chemicals so they could be stored for long periods of time— and a subsequent commercial spin-off.

After the war, the issue of "chemicals in food had become unmanageable," noted G. Edward Damon, a Food and Drug Administration writer, in an article entitled "A Primer On Food Additives," in a 1973 issue of the agency's official publication, *FDA Consumer*.

A Congressional panel, ultimately under the chairmanship of Representative James Delaney of New York, investigated poison in food and out of this came the Pesticide Chemicals Act of 1954, the Food Additives Amendment of 1958 and the Color Additives Amendments of 1960—all tagged onto the Food, Drug and Cosmetic Act of 1938.

But the legislation was still flawed.

On one hand, the "Delaney Clause" became law. It prohibits any level of a cancer-causing substance in food. It declares, "No additive shall be deemed to be safe if it is found to induce cancer when ingested by man or animal." The FDA bitterly fought against the Delaney Clause, FDA officials arguing that cancer should not be singled out among diseases that food additives cause. But Delaney threatened to hold up the entire bill unless the clause remained in it.

For the first time, under the legislation a showing was required that a food additive was safe—but by tests by the manufacturer. As Damon described it, government by providing for manufacturer-testing was showing its "intention . . . not to ban the use of food chemicals but to insure their safety when properly used. All these laws put upon industry the responsibility to prove by scientific research acceptable to the FDA that the substances would be safe as used."

And most importantly, the 1938 law's ban on poisons in food other than what were deemed "unavoidable" or "necessary in production" was altered *to allow poisons* in small doses found not to harm animals.

"This means it is now possible for unlimited numbers of poisons to be injected into foods," charged William Longgood in his book, *The Poisons In Your Food,* published in 1960. He described the legislation as "primarily . . . designed to accommodate industry and protect profits rather than consumers."

Interestingly, although government had begun using "cost-benefit" as a notion in evaluating various risks, the new legislation specifically ordered that no assessment be made of whether additives provided any benefit. "Congress, at the prodding of industry, made clear," noted Damon, "that benefits are not to be considered. The industry feared FDA would refuse to approve any new food additives which provided little benefit over the ones already on the market."

As Dr. Herbert Ley, an FDA commissioner expressed it on his last day of office in 1969: "The thing that bugs me is that the people think the FDA is protecting them—it isn't. What the FDA is doing and what the public thinks it's doing are as different as night and day."

Or as Longgood wrote: "How many more people are dying now or will die in the future because our food laws are designed to protect commercial interests first, and people afterwards? It is generally believed that the public is protected by the Pure Food Law. But it wasn't until the summer of 1958—some fifty-two years after passage of the original law— that Congress finally got around to requiring that chemicals be tested for 'safety' before they could be injected into foods, and then the new law was riddled with so many loopholes that it was largely ineffective as an instrument for consumer protection."

And so, he noted, "virtually every bite of food you eat has been treated with some chemicals somewhere along the line: dyes, bleaches, emulsifiers, antioxidants, preservatives, flavors, buffers, noxious sprays, acidifiers, alkalizers, deodorants, moisteners, drying agents, gases, extenders, thickeners, disinfectants, defoliants, fungicides, neutralizers, sweeteners, anticaking and antifoaming agents, conditioners, curers, hydrolizers, hydrogenators, maturers, fortifiers, and many others."

Indeed, the FDA's line has really not been too different from that of the Chemical Manufacturers Association or the Institute of Food Technologists.

As Damon declared in the *FDA Consumer:*

Can We Get Along Without Additives?

We can get along without food additives, but not as well. Were it not for food additives, we would have to go back to the old concept of bakery freshness—good today, stale tomorrow.

Many of us remember when the cottage cheese separated, cookies dried up in two days, any food with fat or oil in it became rancid, canned vegetables and fruits were soft and mushy, and marshmallows got too hard to toast. Without additives the variety and quality of foods would return to those familiar to grandmother.

The quantities available would definitely be less, and convenience foods would be nonexistent. FDA believes that its work assures the safe use of food additives.

Those "Poisonouschemicals"
Some people have expressed their feelings by coining a term that doesn't actually exist, "poisonouschemicals." If all chemicals are poisonous, then people should stop eating, because all foods are chemicals. Some familiar additives are pure chemicals, such as the potassium iodide in table salt and many familiar vitamins—all essential to man's health.

Expressing foods in chemical terms can be a lengthy job. For example, milk is made of water, 12 fats. 6 proteins. lactose (milk sugar), 9 salts, 7 acids, 3 pigments, 7 enzymes. 18 vitamins, 6 nitrogenous compounds and 3 gases —and the chemical names of these would take another page, at least. Milk is a formidable chemical, but hardly poisonous to most Americans.

Preservatives. There are many kinds, some effective for a particular type of food or against a particular spoilage organism. They are called antioxidants, inhibitors, fungicides, and sequestrants.
Emulsifiers improve the uniformity, fineness of grain, smoothness and body of such foods as bakery goods, ice cream and confectionery products.
Stabilizers and thickeners give that desired smoothness of texture and uniformity of color and flavor to confectioneries, ice creams and other frozen desserts, chocolate milk and artificially sweetened beverages. Commonly used are pectins, vegetable gums and gelatins.
Flavors and flavoring agents represent our largest group of food additives. We are familiar with many, including the spices and liquid derivatives of onion, garlic, cloves and peppermint.

Bleaching agents and maturing agents speed up the aging process which improves the breadmaking quality of flour. Freshly milled flour is yellowish in color and makes very poor bread.
Colors are considered highly important although they do not improve eating qualities. We are so used to a certain color in a specific food that we would refuse to buy and eat it if some other color was present, or the expected color was too pale to look "healthy."

Additives have many other uses, including hardening, drying, leavening, anti-foaming, firming, crisping, anti-sticking, whipping, creaming, clarifying, and sterilizing.

Without these many aids to food processing, today's grocery stores would need a lot less room to sell what foods would be left.

The Job Is Never Done
Food additives are a part of today's modern food technology. The first impetus for Federal control involved Dr. Wiley and his Poison Squad. The second strong push came during and after World War II, when hundreds of new chemicals were suddenly tried and then used to protect and enhance food, particularly for military purposes.

Today, there are thousands of tested and approved food additives. Many are approved only for certain products and in exact amounts. New techniques and improved machinery keep pace with new additives which, if approved by FDA, will further improve our food supply.

And here are segments from a series in 1979 issues of *FDA Consumer* promoting food additives:

More Than You Ever Thought You Would Know About Food Additives

Additives are plentiful—and controversial. They are put into our foods for several reasons. Mostly they are products of modern technology. Because they are so common in today's foods and so controversial, the Food and Drug Administration offers this article and additive index, designed to tell consumers more than they ever thought they would know about additives.

by Phyllis Lehmann

Food additives are so much a part of the American way of eating today that most of us would find it difficult to put together a meal that did not include them.

Take a typical lunch, for example: sandwich, instant soup, gelatin dessert, and a cola drink. The bread has been fortified with vitamins and also contains an additive to keep it fresh. The margarine has been colored pale yellow—or, if you use salad dressing, it has been made with emulsifiers to keep it from "separating." The luncheon meat contains nitrite; the soup, an additive to keep it from becoming rancid; the gelatin, red coloring to make it pretty. Finally, the cola to wash it all down: without coloring, flavoring, sweeteners, or artificial carbonation, the pause that refreshes is, nothing more than plain water!

No wonder many Americans have become concerned. Additives seem to be in everything we eat. Are all these substances good for us? Do they serve a useful purpose, or do they just make money for the food industry?

To help you clarify your own thinking on these questions, let's explore how our present situation came about, and what choices we have.

Food additives are not something new. Humans probably have been tinkering with food since the first caveman killed his first wild boar. Salt was used probably even before recorded history to preserve meat and fish. Herbs and spices have been treasured over the years solely for their capacity to add pizzazz to foods, not to mention their function in a less technological age as a preservative.

Changing lifestyles in this century have resulted in more additives than former generations could have imagined. As Americans moved from farms to cities, there was a need for foods that could be mass produced, distributed over considerable distances, and stored for long periods. The exodus of women from the home into the outside workplace created a demand for more pre-prepared convenience foods. Greater sophistication increased demand for year-round supplies of seasonal products. Greater buying power gave industry a bigger market to please. So today we have a wider variety of foods available—and more additives in all foods—than had ever been known in the past.

The fact that additives are in foods does not please everyone. Many contend that some additives are often dangerous or at least "unnecessary chemicals." The critics note that some additives can cause allergic reactions in some people.

Unnecessary Chemicals was the title of an article in the March 1978 issue of ENVIRONMENT magazine in which the author contended that "many hazardous chemicals (in food and other products) provide consumers with trivial or no benefits at all . . .". The writer, Anita Johnson, an attorney for the Environmental Defense Fund, believes that women shoppers don't want many of the additives. She cited a March 1976 Gallup poll done for RED-BOOK magazine, which "found that 59 percent of the women surveyed said they favored banning food additives used only to improve the appearance of food even if there was no positive evidence of harm."

However, food processors apparently think otherwise and their sales figures would seem to back their thinking. Moreover, the Nation's laws on the subject are designed not to question use of additives but to assure that they are as safe as possible.

By broadest definition, a food additive is any substance that becomes part of a food product when added either directly or indirectly. Today, some 2,800 substances are intentionally added to foods to produce a desired effect. As many as 10,000 other compounds or combinations of compounds find their way into various foods during processing, packaging, or storage. Examples of these unintentional additives include infinitesimal residues of pesticides used to treat crops, minute amounts of drugs fed to animals, and chemical substances that migrate from plastic packaging materials.

Moreover, the Nation's laws on the subject are designed not to question use of additives. . .

More Than You Ever Thought You Would Know About Food Additives... Part II

by Phyllis Lehmann

Time was when there was some credibility to the claims that white bread is not as nutritious as the dark-hued varieties. Not so today. Nevertheless, old notions die hard.

The suspicion that preservatives in bread are the cause of the "cancer epidemic" is not supported by the available scientific evidence. But it's a notion that has considerable life to it.

Is fortifying food tampering with nature? Some critics say it is. They maintain that nutrients synthesized in the laboratory and added during processing are inferior to those present naturally in food. Actually, each vitamin, mineral, or amino acid has a specific molecular structure that is the same whatever the origin of the compound. The body cannot distinguish between a vitamin that occurs naturally in a plant or animal product and the same compound created in a laboratory.

Over the years, a number of common substances have been used to protect foods from microbial action. The oldest is salt, probably used before recorded history, to preserve meat and fish. Sugar has long been used in jams and jellies and to help preserve canned and frozen fruits. Today, such chemicals as sodium propionate and potassium sorbate are used to extend the shelf life of breads, cheeses, syrups, cakes, beverages, mayonnaise, and margarine.

Of the 30 or so chemicals that protect foods from microorganisms, sodium nitrite currently generates the most controversy. A basically garden-variety chemical, nitrite is regularly formed in the body when bacteria act on nitrates, a related group of compounds found in most food and water, or on other nitrogen-containing substances.

Under the Reagan administration, the FDA has been among the targets for "deregulation"—to eliminate or dull what little teeth it has. A major goal: elimination of the Delaney Clause barring any amount of a cancer-causing substance in food.

Dr. Arthur Hull Hayes, Jr., Reagan's commissioner of the FDA, says the "current mandate . . . that if a food additive causes cancer at any dose in any species of animal, it may not be licensed" is "not always flexible enough."

He insists: "It doesn't matter that the incidence of cancer was miniscule or that it occurred only in mice and only at extremely large dosage levels. It doesn't matter that science has changed since 1938, when many of the food laws were passed, or the 1950's, when they were amended."

This same Dr. Hull declared upon taking office:

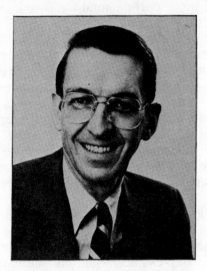

by Arthur Hull Hayes Jr., M.D.
Commissioner of Food and Drugs

Anniversaries are special occasions. They provide an opportunity not only for ceremony but also for reflection and rededication.

As I take over the responsibilities and duties of the Commissioner of Food and Drugs, I reflect on the contributions made by the first "commissioner," Dr. Harvey Washington Wiley.

Dr. Wiley is aptly called the "father" of the Food and Drugs Act of 1906. He fought for a quarter of a century for a safer food and drug supply. As chief of the Bureau of Chemistry—predecessor of today's Food and Drug Administration—Dr. Wiley directed the first years of enforcement under the Food and Drugs Act.

I believe that Dr. Harvey Wiley, could he see his legacy, would be pleased. It remains for us to remember his great tradition and to carry it forward as we go about our work.

There is a key flaw in the argument of Hayes and other opponents of the Delaney Clause that cancer occurring in test animals when a high dose of a substance is administered is not indicative of what might happen to humans.

As Anita Johnson of the Environmental Defense Fund has explained: "Large doses are essential for animal studies. They compensate for the short lifespan of animals relative to humans and for the fast metabolization and excretion of chemicals by animals compared to humans . . . Low-dose animal studies would not be valuable in detecting cancer-causing chemicals, as industry well knows when it advocates using low doses only. High-dose animal studies are considered by cancer experts to be highly predictive of human harm."

On the behest of the Reagan administration, Senator Orrin Hatch, a Republican from Utah, has been a leader in Congress pushing to end the Delaney Clause, with a "food safety reform bill."

The Society of the Plastics Industry, the American Meat Institute and the National Soft Drink Association, three of the trade groups involved in lobbying efforts for this 1981 bill sent a letter to members of Congress declaring that "although the food safety laws have basically worked well to assure that the American food supply is safe, varied and affordable, the increasing disparity between those laws and current scientific knowledge has led to an increasing strain on their implementation."

The Hatch bill has been battled by consumer and health organizations including the Coalition for Safe Food, led by the Washington-based Community Nutrition Institute.

At one point, Senator Albert Gore, a Democrat from Tennessee, said the Hatch bill "has the makings of a fraud about to be perpetrated on the American people."

Then Gore came up with his own bill in 1982, largely fashioned by an aide who was a former administrator with the U.S. Department of Agriculture. It, too, would replace the Delaney Clause. Ellen Haas, consumer director of the Community Nutrition Institute, calls it "little more than a re-Hatched version of the industry wish list that was introduced last year."

Different administrations and political parties vary in degree but, as usual, in the end the loyalty of most of those in American government to the producers of poison is a bipartisan affair.

The Environmental Protection Agency, created in 1970 to be the main American government agency to deal with those who poison the environment, is a prime example of this.

EPA writer Truman Temple related in a 1979 issue of *EPA Journal* that the agency emanated from "the most active period" for U.S. legislation dealing with pollution.

"Measures enacted by Congress during this period," he noted, "have been prompted by widespread concern over environmental damage, by the consumer protection movement, by lawsuits, and by advances in medicine that stressed the need for preventive steps to shield the public from harmful chemicals, rather than costly clean-up activity after the damage has been done. Part of this philosophy reflected a shift in emphasis within the medical profession in dealing with cancer. Many physicians and research professionals felt that more emphasis should be placed on keeping carcinogens out of man's environment rather than on the 'cancer cure' approach."

Laws that the EPA was to administer were the Federal Insecticide, Fungicide and Rodenticide Act of 1972, the Safe Drinking Water Act of 1974, the Resource Conservation and Recovery Act of 1976 and the Toxic Substances Control Act of 1976.

Hugh B. Kaufman has been there from the beginning. Once he was the EPA's chief investigator for toxic waste but, having warned in speeches, interviews and Congressional testimony that the government, in fact, has been doing little or nothing to protect citizens from the dangers of toxic chemicals, he has been relegated to a nonpolicy job.

"If I were a Russian spy and wanted to poison the American people," he told the House Subcommittee on Commerce, Transportation and Tourism in 1982, he wouldn't change the U.S. toxic waste program "one iota." He said, "I couldn't plan a better way of doing it than the way the government is handling the hazardous waste issue."

"Peoples' air and water is being poisoned and the government continues to lie to them about how they are being protected," he told the panel.

Back at his desk as assistant to the head of EPA's Hazard-ous Site Control Division to which he has been shunted, Kauf-man is saying that the EPA was "less under the thumb" of polluting industries in its first several years. The agency's initial administrators were able to "deflect" pressures.

Kaufman notes that William Ruckelshaus, EPA's first ad-ministrator, had a "power base in the Indiana Republican Party. He was assistant U.S. attorney general and very well-liked and respected by a broad spectrum of the limousine liberal/power elite of the country, both Republicans and Democrats." So whether it was pressure from the White House, the Office of Management and Budget "or whatever," he was able "to keep the agency a little more on the straight and narrow."

The second EPA administrator, Russell Train, was "a for-mer tax judge, very well-connected in Washington with the environmental groups" and the "power elite on the Hill, a man of substance, of character" who could parry pressure, too, says Kaufman.

It was under President Carter that "the character of the leadership changed" and EPA "became more under the thumb" of industry.

Carter appointed Douglas Costle as EPA administrator and Barbara Blum as his deputy. Costle, says Kaufman, was "really a junior kind of guy with no constituency" and Blum's only "claim to fame is that she was a good political hack." She had been deputy manager of Carter's first campaign.

At that point "the pressures of industry on the agency got stronger. And, of course," says Kaufman, with the Reagan administration, "there's no doubt in any one's mind where they're coming from."

Mrs. Gorsuch "had no constituency," he adds, "other than Joseph Coor's," the ultra-conservative Colorado beer-producer who was "her Godfather. Coor's money put her in political office; she was part of that club." She "came in strictly as a political hack just working her way up career-wise."

The appointment of top officials of polluting industries as top administrators of EPA under the Reagan administration "certainly does have an effect," says Kaufman. But the differences from the Carter administration are nevertheless not marked.

Explains Kaufman: "For example, here we have Assistant Administrator Rita Lavelle who's responsible for toxic waste, both Superfund and regulation, who before this was the PR director of Aerojet-General, a major toxic waste polluter. And, in fact, Aerojet-General is responsible for major pollution cases both in northern California and in Riverside, California. The first one was a groundwater contamination case where they wiped out a drinking water supply of a large number of homes and it was Lavelle's job to PR Aerojet out of that fix. Then she was put in charge of the regulatory system. But in this job, even though she's cutting it on industry's side, she's certainly no more, no less protective than the Carter appointee, Chris Beck, who did not come from that background. The difference is in her rhetoric. Her rhetoric is much more pro-industry whereas Beck's rhetoric was a little softer, but the culmination down the line of what's actually promulgated, not proposed or thrown up as red herrings in speeches, but actually promulgated is basically the same.

"Gorsuch is very cunning," Kaufman continues. "She is good at muddying up the issues and it's much more oppressive especially for technical people inside the organization. "I'm not sure that what came out the door" in the Reagan administration's "final regulatory package is any worse than would have come out the door in the Carter administration. It's just that their tactics are a little bit seedier or sleazier in terms of getting their way.

In the area of his specialty, toxic waste, those who generate toxic waste "want to transfer the liability of these wastes off their property into the public's backyard at the cheapest possible costs."

So government writes regulations accordingly, from administration to administration, he says. "The tactics that an administration would use on the technical people to impose their will would change, basically as a function of style. The style of the Carter people was that they were a little more gentlemanly. They weren't as much street-type politicos."

He agrees that in some instances poisoning can and should

just be ordered stopped. He notes the California move "to prohibit certain wastes from going to landfills where a technology has been demonstrated that's clearly much safer than landfills." Such poisons simply would not be allowed to be dumped in the ground.

But, says Kaufman, he sees regulation appropriate in an area like "setting limits for peoples' drinking water" when it becomes contaminated by "toxic chemicals, which invariably will happen; we can't close our eyes to the fact that some water supplies are going to be wiped out. You do need some vehicle to measure what will trigger a response to get an alternative water supply and what would not, and this requires regulation. Even though the government may not be the best or the perfect vehicle for developing those kinds of regulations, at least the public has a shot if government does it. If it's merely done by industry consensus . . . the public is really frozen out, and the chance of the light of day seeing the deliberation process is much less. So I don't know of any other way to handle that type of situation other than through a government regulatory body, bringing in scientists, and also having the chance of the light and day hitting it through a democracy-type operation."

He thus feels there is not "one sole answer; I think you have to have a mix."

As to keeping the would-be protectors protecting, Kaufman sees "two important factors. You must have the person in the White House being from a different party than the people on Capitol Hill, so you have that check and balance. And the second thing is that the news media has a tremendous responsibility to cover in more detail these issues, casting the light of day on them in proportion to the importance of the issue to the society."

He speaks of making a check of a "data bank" for media reports on "key deliberative actions that occur that affect everyone's life." Pollution of drinking water, "which is pretty damn important, it affects a lot of people," would be found to have gotten far less attention "in the national media than Nancy Reagan's dishes and clothes," he declares. "You'll find no comparison. And the effect of Nancy Reagan's dishes and clothes is absolutely minimal to the life of the American people compared to the drinking water supply."

As a result of Kaufman's outspoken honesty, EPA investigators have shadowed him on vacation trips, recorded a public appearance, and bugged his office phone. "It's harassment," says Kaufman, with "secret police tactics." During the Carter administration, the man who was once the government's chief investigator for toxic waste was transferred to a non-policy staff job, and the Reagan administration has made sure he stays there.

But Kaufman says he will not be silenced. His commitment to speak the truth about the government's countenance of pollution began when he first began investigating toxic waste dumps.

"Once you talk face to face with people who live near a toxic dump, you're never the same," he explains. "They can't get safe drinking water, can't sell their homes and are total prisoners."

Kaufman says: "We're on a collision course with wiping out our water supplies in 20 to 30 years and the Reagan administration is fiddling. The people in the EPA now are a destruction crew. They're cutting the staff, slashing the budget and tripling the red tape. The result is that nothing gets done."

William Sanjour is another EPA insider with the guts to speak out. He notes that it isn't that "a lot of people don't agree" with what Kaufman and he "are saying, but they're certainly not about to fight the organization actively."

Sanjour came to the EPA in 1974, and was "quite enthusiastic when I came here. I don't come from an environmentalist background; I come from a consulting background, as someone who likes to solve problems." He began investigating the issue of hazardous waste, not knowing whether "it was a serious problem or not. I spent a lot of your money studying it for many years and found out it is a very serious problem, but there are solutions. And I was instrumental in getting the legislation [on hazardous waste] written and passed.

"I thought we would settle down then to start implementing but instead of implementing, it's gone every way but right," he notes.

As he told the Senate Subcommittee on Oversight of Government Management in 1979:

STATEMENT OF
WILLIAM SANJOUR
CHIEF, HAZARDOUS WASTE IMPLEMENTATION BRANCH,
STATE PROGRAMS AND RESOURCE RECOVERY DIVISION
ENVIRONMENTAL PROTECTION AGENCY

BEFORE THE
SUBCOMMITTEE ON OVERSIGHT OF GOVERNMENT MANAGEMENT
COMMITTEE ON GOVERNMENTAL AFFAIRS
UNITED STATES SENATE

August 1, 1979

Mr. Chairman and Members of the Subcommittee, I am
William Sanjour, Chief of the Hazardous Waste Implementation
Branch of the Environmental Protection Agency (EPA). I was
formerly Chief of the Assessment and Technology Branch in
the Hazardous Waste Management Division.

I am here at the request of the Subcommittee to testify
on what I know of the development of regulations for hazardous
waste under the Resource Conservation and Recovery Act of
1976 (RCRA). My testimony will focus on the process by
which the proposed regulations were arrived at, particularly
with regard to EPA upper management actions and directives
that affected the development of the regulations. In my
opinion, those actions and directives reflect EPA mismanagement
and departure from the statutory mandate and are a major
contributor to the delay in promulgating the RCRA regulations.

It was clear from the earliest days that hazardous
waste regulation did not have the support of our upper
management or the Administration. For example:

o   The Administration in 1975 instructed EPA officials
      and officials from other agencies to testify
      against passage of hazardous waste legislation
      when it was being considered by Congress.

o   During the same period, EPA upper management
      urged the Hazardous Waste Management Division to
      "jawbone" with industry rather than seek regulatory
      authority over hazardous waste.

o   When RCRA passed, the Administration did not ask
      Congress for sufficient resources to implement it.

o   The development of hazardous waste regulations
      was made subordinate within EPA to the clean water program
      which was responsible for producing much of the
      hazardous waste.

He testified: "In general, efforts were made to downplay the
need for hazardous waste management."

In 1978, he reported, two years after passage of the Resource Conservation and Recovery Act despite the EPA re-
sistance, "we were informed by our management that because
of pressure from the White House," steps were to be taken to
weaken the regulations to be issued for the law.

They had not yet been issued because of "a lack of leadership and will" of the EPA "upper management."

(1) We were directed not to rely on objective charac-
      teristics and test protocols to identify hazardous
      waste, but to rely instead on lists of specific
      industrial processes to be regulated. It was felt that use
      of characteristics put too great an economic

burden on industry for testing. We were so
informed, despite all the research we had invested
in, despite the fact that RCRA doesn't allow for
economic factors to be taken into account in defining
a hazardous waste, and despite the fact that the
initial cost of regulating hazardous waste disposal
properly is far less than the ultimate economic,
health and social costs of not regulating and of
later having to clean up the land;

(2)   We were to avoid regulating hazardous waste from
the oil and gas industry, electric power companies,
and other large industries;

(3)   We were to avoid regulating the hazardous waste
from industries or municipalities which have water
discharge permits under the Clean Water Act.

And, testified Sanjour:

We were also told to stop looking for hazardous waste
disposal sites which posed an imminent hazard to public
health, to delay getting out the regulations while we re-
studied all possible options, and to keep all this from the
public.

He declared:

As a result of the news stories about leaking dump
sites such as Love Canal and the "Valley of the Drums,"
the focus has been on what to do about these sites,

whereas the infinitely more important issue from the standpoint of public health is what to do to prevent such sites in the future.

The Administration is moving away from doing things which protect the environment in favor of doing things which take care of the consequences of not doing the things which protect the environment. To illustrate how far this has gone, we are spending millions in Federal funds to clean up Love Canal in Niagara Falls but we have dropped from our proposed hazardous waste regulations those very wastes which we are cleaning up. "Taking care of the consequences of the failure to protect the environment" is not the same thing as "protecting the environment". Nor is it a substitute for environmental protection. Therefore it is a sham to refer to superfund as "environmental legislation" when in fact it is really disaster relief.

In conclusion, Sanjour testified:

First and most obvious, there is no substitute for enthusiasm and the will to do the job you're charged with. In my opinion, EPA and the Administration do not want to regulate industrial disposal of hazardous waste. Unless this lack of will and attitude is changed, any money or positions added to EPA's budget for hazardous waste management is wasted and could be counterproductive.

. . . EPA and the Administration do not want to regulate industrial disposal of hazardous waste.

In 1982, Sanjour was saying that he has found the Carter and Reagan administrations "about the same" in protecting people from pollution.

"The one difference," he notes, "is the Carter administration had an environmental constituency, which the Reagan administration doesn't. The Carter administration, at least, had to keep an environmental front up, so what they did was spend a lot of money on the environment. You see, they had to serve two masters: they had industry which they were trying to placate, on one hand, and they had environmentalists they wanted to placate. The way they solved their problem was to spend an awful lot of money on the environment but see to it that it didn't do anything. Spending the money satisfied the environmentalists. They think you can solve problems by throwing money at them. That's why Superfund was invented, by the way. When Love Canal blew up in peoples' faces and became a very publicized event, the agency's response, I would have thought, would be, 'Well, all right, let us now implement the regulations which will prevent this problem in the future.' They didn't do that. They continued to sabotage the regulations. What they did was invent a huge Superfund to clean up the waste instead of preventing it. In other words, if you're faced with an outbreak of polio, what they're doing is buying more iron lungs instead of investing in the vaccine. Meanwhile, they're sabotaging the vaccine program. They turn around and invent a huge program of building hospitals and iron lungs. And that satisfied the environmentalists. It was a trick. It made the environmentalists think, 'Look, we're spending a lot of money in cleaning up waste so we must be doing something good.' It satisfied the waste disposal industry because they made a fortune out of Superfund. What Superfund does is to take waste from one landfill and move it to another landfill. And they get paid for it. In fact, the very same people who Superfund was moving against were in some cases actually getting paid to move the waste around. They pay a small fine for their previous pollution and make a fortune for moving it somewhere else."

The federal government "just makes matters worse and they spend a lot of money making them worse," Sanjour goes on. "The one thing I have to say for Reagan is that at least he doesn't spend a hell of a lot of money making matters worse. He makes them worse but he's cheap with the money because he doesn't have an environmental constituency; that's basically it."

Sanjour says he now regards the situation as "hopeless." In the field of landfills, for example, what EPA has done "is to institutionalize landfills. The worst possible way of disposing of waste has now been institutionalized. That's the upshot of the federal regulations."

Polluting has been brought "under federal auspices." He cites the case of landfills where the owner of a dump, who before could be sued for the damage it caused, now as a result of government action is largely immune from liability. "Since the federal government got involved," says Sanjour, "we have passed a law which makes the owner of a landfill, five years after he closes it no longer able to be sued for liability for that landfill. In other words, the liability provisions of Common Law have been removed by Act of Congress."

"Does that encourage people to be responsible or irresponsible?" asks Sanjour. "Since by Act of Congress, they can no longer be held responsible for what they do, does that encourage them to be responsible?"

"We have," he continues, "written standards for hazardous waste landfills which basically allow existing landfills to go on doing what they have been doing. But before, when they were doing it at least they could be sued by somebody that they were damaging. Now, since they are in compliance with all federal standards, even while they're operating they can't be sued."

He says that EPA "put in a camouflage of requiring an insurance provision for landfills. EPA made a big to-do about that. First they dropped the provision, then there was a big hue and cry about the agency dropping the provision, so they reinstitated the insurance provision. The true provision is that at the first sign of any trouble the insurance company can cancel—which means, you're insured for as long as there's no trouble. If there's any trouble, there's no insurance."

"I can go on and on about these regulations," says Sanjour. "They basically institutionalized the worst possible practices."

And, "there are many alternatives" to landfills," he stresses. "There is no hazardous waste that need ever be landfilled" and "in fact, landfilling hazardous wastes is probably the most expensive thing you can do." But "it's just that the guy who dumps the stuff in the landfill" can get off seemingly cheap. "The taxpayer has to pay." For a fraction of the ultimate public cost of dealing with hazardous waste dumped in a landfill, the generator of the poison could eliminate it by alternative means, says Sanjour. By permitting dumping instead, "you're saving the guy who generates the waste a nickel and spending $10 to save him a nickel."

Sanjour says he has become "completely distrustful of the federal government." As to a political solution to the massive problem of poison pollution, he asks: "What makes you think there's a solution?"

As Sanjour wrote to Lois Gibbs, whose family was forced from their home at Love Canal due to waste dumping there and who went on to head the Citizen's Clearinghouse for Hazardous Wastes:

UNITED STATES ENVIRONMENTAL PROTECTION AGENCY
WASHINGTON, D.C. 20460

February 26, 1982

OFFICE OF
SOLID WASTE AND EMERGENCY RESPONSE

Mrs. Lois Gibbs
P.O. Box 7097
Arlington, VA 22207

Dear Mrs. Gibbs:

In response to your inquiry about citizens fears regarding new technology state-of-the-art hazardous waste landfills, I have drawn up what in my personal opinion is a good analogy of the situation.

Suppose there were an airplane manufacturer who had a long history of making planes that crashed. And suppose he came out with a new model which he claimed was "state-of-the-art" and guaranteed not to crash. But suppose you found out that no insurance company would insure the plane. And suppose you further found out that the aircraft manufacturer had been lobbying Congress for years and has succeeded in getting a law passed that "in the event even today's best state-of-the-art technology does manage to fail sometime in the future" the aircraft manufacturer could not be held responsible. In addition, suppose there was an independent study of some of the few such planes actually flying and they were found to have cracks in them. Would you fly that plane?

Well the people who manage hazardous waste have a long history of building landfills that leak and pollute and endanger public health. (80% of the EPA list of the 115 priority sites for "superfund" clean-up were legitimate hazardous waste landfills.) Nevertheless industry spokesman say that today's high technology state-of-the-art hazardous waste landfills bear no more relationship to those old chemical dumps than a modern office building bears to a tarpaper shack. In spite of this, no insurance company will insure these state-of-the-art facilities. And the hazardous waste management industry lobbied Congress for years until it got legislation which five years after closure, transfers liability for the landfill to the taxpayer and removes the citizens right to sue the landfill operator for damages. Furthermore, a recent study at Princeton University of four new stateof-the-art hazardous waste landfills in New Jersey shows evidence of leakage.

Is it therefore unreasonable for the public to be wary about such landfills?

Very truly yours,

William Sanjour
Chief, Hazardous Waste Implementation Branch
Office of Solid Waste

Very much like the FDA, the story of the EPA has been one of promise not fulfilled, or PR not performance—of a sell-out.

Jacqueline Warren is an attorney for the 45,000-member Natural Resources Defense Council which has closely monitored what EPA has done—or more accurately, failed to do—in implementing the Toxic Substances Control Act (TSCA).

As she told the House Subcommittee on Energy, Environment and Natural Resources in 1981:

> TSCA was passed in response to repeated disclosures about the severe adverse health, environmental and economic damage inflicted by such widely used substances as PCBs, kepone, vinyl chloride, PBBs and asbestos, to name but a few. The Act was intended to remedy the lack of legal authority to prevent such problems from arising, or to deal adequately with them after the fact of injury or serious risk was established.
>
> The clearly-stated overriding purpose of TSCA is to prevent unreasonable risks of injury to health and the environment from exposure to toxic substances. The basic objectives of the law, as set forth in section 2, are that adequate data on the effects of chemicals should be developed by those who produce them; that EPA should have adequate authority to regulate chemical substances which present an unreasonable risk of injury to health and the environment; and that undue or unnecessary burdens on commerce and innovation should be avoided in "fulfilling the primary purpose of the Act to assure that such innovation and commerce in chemical substances and mixtures do not present an unreasonable risk of injury to health or the environment".
>
> To achieve these purposes, Congress provided EPA the authority to require that chemicals be tested to determine whether they are hazardous; to restrict or even prohibit their manufacture and use in appropriate circumstances; and to screen new chemicals to identify potential "bad actors" before, rather than long after, their entry into commerce. Yet, EPA's record in moving to identify and abate chemical hazards during the four years TSCA has been on the books is noteworthy primarily for its failures rather than for its successes.

The three principal regulatory authorities established by TSCA, *i.e.*, to require testing, to screen new chemicals, and to control chemicals found to pose unreasonable risks of injury to health or the environment have been implemented either slowly, poorly, or rarely. Moreover, the new Administration appears to be focusing its efforts on finding ways for the chemical industry to avoid complying with the few TSCA requirements that are now in effect. Furthermore, the regulated industry is playing a predominant role in the effort to develop exemptions from TSCA and to find ways around the requirements of the statute. At the same time, the public is entirely excluded from the process.

This assessment of EPA's performance is not cavalierly made. Despite repeated criticisms of EPA by organizations such as NRDC, the EPA Administrator's own Toxic Substances Advisory Committee, and members of Congress, it is clear the mandate of TSCA is not being fulfilled. Now even the relatively few strides made in the past to control the introduction of new toxic substances into commerce, and to begin testing widely-used chemicals suspected of being toxic, may be reversed.

She noted that as of 1981:
• EPA "has not yet required a single chemical to be tested" and instead has accepted "voluntary testing proposals" of chemical manufacturers.

• EPA "is not accomplishing the stated objective of TSCA that the health and environmental effects of a substance be determined before commercial production begins."

• The agency is "rarely" using its power under the TSCA to direct that warnings for certain products be made, that there be limits and restrictions on use and outright prohibitions.

• EPA "has failed to act against" toxic chemicals designated by the EPA staff for "high priority regulatory action."

Said Ms. Warren: "Four years after TSCA was enacted, the chemical industry in the United States generally appears to be conducting business as usual, and continuing to use the workplace, the general public and the environment as a testing laboratory for determining the adverse effects of their products."

EPA is a "classic illustration of the 'captive agency' syndrome, in which the industry exercises undue influence over the regulatory agency to the detriment of the public at large." She summed up:

> In the area of toxic substances control, the frequently voiced assertion that we have done enough and should now cut back, has a very hollow ring. In contrast to various other federal programs, we are only now at the very beginning of the effort to come to grips with the problems posed by the marketing, use and disposal of toxic chemicals whose hazards are not identified until after the fact of health, environmental, and economic damage.
>
> TSCA was enacted in response to a strong public demand for a basic institutional change in the way chemicals are developed and introduced so that the potential PCBs of the future will be identified in the laboratory rather than in medical records or in monetary losses caused by contamination incidents. Congress' intention that TSCA would begin to remedy such problems has not yet been carried out and the problems caused by toxic substances are still with us. Unfortunately, the up-coming drastic budget and personnel cuts at EPA, coupled with the Agency's apparent willingness to accede to virtually all of the chemical industry's wishes, portend even less effective implementation of TSCA than the EPA's prior record demonstrates.

Under the Reagan administration, the EPA—as derelict as it had become before—took a deeper dive.

A grouping of some of America's most prominent environmental organizations—Friends of the Earth, Environmental Defense Fund, Sierra Club, National Audubon Society, Natural Resources Defense Council, Environmental Action, Defenders of Wildlife, Environmental Policy Center, Solar Lobby, Wilderness Society—in March 1982 issued this *Indictment:*

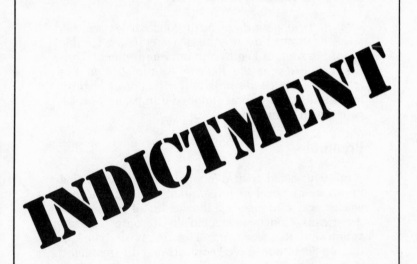

The Case Against
the Reagan Environmental Record

Clean Air • Clean Water • Hazardous Wastes • Toxics • Strip Mining • Public Lands • National Forests • National Parks • Wilderness • Endangered Species OCS • Coal Leasing • Nuclear • Solar • Energy Conservation • Synfuels • International • Regulatory Reform • Council on Environmental Quality •

On the issue of the poisoning of the environment, the *Indictment* included these points:

Hazardous Wastes

Millions of pounds of hazardous wastes are disposed of every day in America creating a terrible hazard to human health and our environment. During the past year the Reagan Administration has retreated from its responsibility to control hazardous dumps, clean up abandoned dumps, and prosecute illegal dumpers.

Preamble

In 1976, faced with overwhelming evidence that improper disposal of huge quantities of hazardous wastes was endangering the health of millions of Americans, Congress enacted the Resource Conservation and Recovery Act. The Act is designed to impose "cradle to grave" controls on "the treatment, storage, transportation, and disposal of hazardous wastes which have adverse effects on health and the environment . . .." Some 130 billion pounds of hazardous wastes are created each year. The goal of the hazardous waste law is to asure safe, tightly regulated handling and disposal of newly created wastes.

In 1980 Congress enacted legislation creating a "Superfund" to provide for cleanup of abandoned dumpsites and dangerous spills of toxic materials and to facilitate compensation of victims. The law imposes a tax on chemical producers, the revenues from which are placed in a fund to be used exclusively to clean up dumps and spills. The intent of Congress was that EPA aggressively seek to compel the responsible parties to complete the required cleanup and, failing that, use Superfund resources to do so.

Charges

From Love Canal to the Valley of the Drums, the need for action is urgently apparent, yet during the past year EPA Administrator Anne Gorsuch and other officials of the Agency have made it unmistakably clear to polluters that hazardous waste controls are being undone.

Loosening Controls on Wastes.

- Shortly after Gorsuch took office, enforcement actions against illegal dumpers came to a halt. Enforcement staff are not even permitted to request information from suspected violators without top-level headquarters approval.
- Regulations to control incineration and surface storage of wastes, required by law to be issued by October 1978, were finally promulgated in January 1981. Gorsuch suspended implementation of these regulations for existing facilities in July 1981 and three months later proposed to withdraw them.
- The law also required regulations for the disposal of hazardous wastes in landfills to be issued by October 1978. EPA planned to get them out in 1981, but Gorsuch, ignoring an outstanding court order, has delayed them.
- Financial responsibility rules designed to assure that firms handling hazardous wastes have the necessary resources to protect the public and pay for damage or injuries resulting from spills, fires, and explosions were issued in January 1981. Gorsuch postponed these rules until April 1982 and has indicated she will suspend them altogether.
- In February 1981, without notice or public comment, Gorsuch suspended the prohibition against burial of liquid wastes in drums, the practice that created Love Canal. The public reaction to the suspension was so strong that EPA was forced to reimpose the ban. However, Gorsuch still proposes to permit the burial of liquid wastes in drums in 25 percent of the area of a landfill.
- In negotiations with industry attorneys in a pending litigation, EPA agreed to weaken permitting requirements for hazardous waste facilities. Facilities may now expand up to 50 percent without having to meet federal requirements.
- In March 1982 EPA deferred reporting requirements for hazardous waste generators. This action pre-

vents citizens from obtaining information about local dumps, impedes enforcement, and deprives EPA of data needed to develop effective regulations.

- Gorsuch has proposed to slash the funds available to states and EPA Regional offices to implement and enforce hazardous waste requirements.

Delaying Implementation of Superfund.

- EPA has listed 115 of the most dangerous dumpsites around the nation. Legal action had been taken against 20 before Gorsuch took office. Since then the EPA enforcement section's major action has been to write letters to invite those responsible for creating the remaining dumps in to talk.
- The Superfund legislation required EPA to develop by June 1981 a National Contingency Plan to guide the search for and cleanup of dangerous sites and to prepare to respond to emergencies such as spills and explosions. A plan was finally proposed in March 1982. The proposal is so vague as to provide no guarantee that Superfund resources and authority will be used to clean up any site. The plan implies that EPA cares more about saving money than cleaning up sites to protect human health.
- In the first use of its Superfund authority, after a toxic dump site in Santa Fe Springs, California, caught fire in July 1981, top EPA officials quickly negotiated a private settlement with one of the responsible parties. The settlement limited the company's cleanup responsibility instead of requiring the cleanup to continue until the hazard was removed. It also *committed EPA to testify on behalf of the company in any subsequent lawsuit against it* arising from the dump and the fire.
- To direct the Superfund effort, Gorsuch has appointed Rita M. Lavelle, public affairs specialist for Aero Jet Liquid Rocket, a company that has, according to EPA, the third worst pollution record in the state of California, including a massive release of arsenic, phenols, sulfates, and a variety of carcinogens into unlined ponds.

The result of these actions is to increase the public health risk from hazardous wastes, as earth, air, surface and groundwater continue to be contaminated. The result is to undercut those responsible industries that have invested in safe waste disposal technologies, and to destroy the credibility EPA had sought to build, enabling it to convince communities across the nation they could safely allow new, regulated waste disposal facilities to be built. The Administration's retreat increases the likelihood of a new Love Canal.

Water Quality

The water that sustains our nation, our rivers, lakes, and underground aquifers, is threatened by sewage, sediments, and toxic chemicals. The law says the discharge of pollutants into the nation's waters must end by 1985. The Administration has chosen to abandon that goal and seeks to weaken the Clean Water Act.

Preamble

Water pollution affects us all. There are over 100,000 dischargers of industrial wastewater in the United States. Waters in every state in the nation are affected by industrial discharges.

Pollution from municipal sewage is even more prevalent. Runoff from city streets and rural lands adds still more pollution to streams, lakes, and coastal waters.

The water we drink may be unsafe. The General Accounting Office recently reported that there were 146,000 violations of safe drinking water standards across the nation in 1980 alone. Fisheries are being destroyed. Industrial discharges of kepone interrupted commercial fishing in Virginia's rich James River, and PCBs did the same to the Hudson River. Swimming, boating, and agriculture are affected.

The Clean Water Act, passed in 1972 and strengthened in 1977, directs the Environmental Protection Agency to develop and enforce rules to achieve the goal of "fishable and swimmable" waters by 1983 and the elimination of *all discharge* of pollutants by 1985. Both the Act and an outstanding court order require EPA to set rules to control the discharge of toxic water pollutants.

The Safe Drinking Water Act was passed in 1974 in response to evidence that the drinking water of many Americans was laced with dangerous chemicals ranging from asbestos to vinyl chloride. Ground water, which provides drinking water for half our citizens, has been contaminated in many places across the nation.

The Safe Drinking Water Act requires EPA to set minimum drinking water quality standards to protect human health and to establish rules to prevent the injection of contaminants into underground aquifers.

Progress has been made in improving water quality. Overall, further deterioration of surface waters seems to have ceased—which is progress, considering that our population and industrial activity are rising. There are numerous individual success stories. Rivers such as the Savannah, the Hudson, the Naugatuck, the Detroit, the Connecticut, and many others showed remarkable improvement. But control of toxic chemical pollution is still at a primitive stage. Ground water pollution is a special worry. It is not well monitored; yet there is mounting evidence that wells from Gray, Maine, to the San Gabriel Valley in California are being polluted by toxic chemicals. Once those chemicals get into ground water, they are terribly difficult and costly to remove.

A huge job remains to protect drinking water sources and achieve the "fishable and swimmable" goal.

Charges

The Reagan Administration has begun to implement policies that will not only halt progress but threatens to cause declines in water quality. Especially alarming is the Administration's retreat on control of toxic pollutants, which affect both surface and groundwaters and make water unfit for drinking and for aquatic life.

Retreating from Control of Toxics. During the past year, the Reagan Administration has

- Suspended the entire national pretreatment program for over one year and suspended critical portions of that program indefinitely. The purpose of the pretreatment program is to curtail toxic discharges into municipal treatment plants by over 60,000 industrial sources.
- Delayed the national program for setting toxic effluent limits on industrial discharges from tens of thousands of sources. Since January 1981, EPA has not issued a single regulation to limit toxic discharges, but has twice requested extensions in court-ordered deadlines. If granted, the delays would extend deadlines from 1981 to mid–1984—resulting in tens of millions of pounds of inadequately treated toxic chemical discharges yearly.
- Sought to escape from its court-ordered responsibility to clean up toxic "hot spots" of chemical pollution. Those are specific locations where even the best available technology will not be sufficient to protect human health and water quality. EPA has done virtually nothing to address this problem.
- Sought to escape from its court-ordered duty to identify dangerous toxic water pollutants that will not be controlled by regulations under development in the Agency.
- Proposed to amend the Clean Water Act by adding variances and deadline extensions to the Act's uniform national toxic cleanup requirements. Those amendments would seriously delay cleanup, add tremendous burdens to state permitting authorities, and ultimately fail to control toxic discharges because of lack of data and scientific methods.
- Decided not to impose new, stricter limits on toxic discharges in revised permits for thousands of industrial dischargers, who will thus be allowed delays in adopting best available technology. Instead of

using the Agency's authority to issue, case by case, permits with stricter toxics limitations than those now in existence, EPA has decided to wait until nationally uniform standards are promulgated—even if it takes 2–3 more years to develop those rules. Of course, the permitting budget was cut accordingly.

• Weakened the standards designed to protect aquifers and eliminated protections against injections of hazardous wastes.

• Failed to develop permanent drinking water quality standards that protect against toxic organic contamination.

Relaxing Other Water Quality Requirements. The Reagan Administration also has

• Developed a regulation (soon to be proposed) that would significantly relax treatment requirements for municipalities. EPA plans to "redefine" the requirement of secondary treatment so that the horrible noncompliance rate by cities suddenly will disappear.

• Developed a regulation (soon to be proposed) that would assist those states wishing to use their waterways for waste transport. In effect, the regulation would encourage states to downgrade their water quality standards, instead of enforcing the Act's national goal of fishable, swimmable water quality.

Toxic Substances

Progress in controlling toxic chemicals that threaten public health and the environment has been disappointingly slow. Now even the little that has been achieved is unravelling. Under the Reagan Administration, EPA's attention is focused on easing requirements on industry, not on increasing protection for the public.

Preamble

Industrial chemicals are pervasive in our world. There are over 40,000 chemicals produced or used in the United States. Ten to twenty new chemical compounds enter the stream of commerce every week. Manmade chemicals are a part of virtually all commercial products used today.

Many chemicals are benign, but some are extraordinarily dangerous, even in tiny quantities. Some cause cancer, birth defects, heart and lung disease, and a host of other ailments. Because the damage they do may take years, even decades, to show up in humans, people often suffer long exposure to hazardous chemicals before their effects are fully known. Vinyl chloride was widely used for many years— despite laboratory tests showing it caused cancer in animals—before we learned that it causes human cancer. Asbestos was used in talcum powder, wallboard, hair dryers, brake linings, and many other products for decades before epidemiological studies definitively showed it is a human carcinogen. Animal studies implicating asbestos as a carcinogen had been done much earlier.

Because of these tragedies in which humans have served as guinea pigs, and because of the proven ability of positive animal testing to predict effects in humans, the federal government established cancer policies which treat animal data as a sufficient basis for regulation. This established policy rejects the view that human evidence ("counting dead bodies") is necessary to initiate protective regulation.

The Toxic Substances Control Act (TSCA) was enacted in 1976 to assure that "innovation and commerce in chemical substances and mixtures do not present an unreasonable risk of injury to health or the environment." TSCA authorizes EPA to require testing of certain existing chemicals to determine whether they are hazardous; to restrict or prohibit the manufacture of chemicals that pose an unreasonable risk to human health; and to screen new chemicals to identify potential "bad actors" before, rather than long after, human beings are exposed to them.

TSCA is a complicated law, and the Carter Administration moved very slowly in carrying it out. It did make a useful beginning, preparing several rules that require manufacturers to test highly suspicious chemicals and proposing quality standards for the data industry submits.

Charges

The Reagan Administration has cancelled the slow progress made so far under TSCA to identify and control toxic chemicals. It has made a dangerous decision, in defiance of the overwhelming weight of scientific opinion, not to accept animal test data alone as presumptive evidence that a chemical is a human carcinogen. It is negotiating with industry on controversial chemicals behind closed doors, with the public and impartial scientists excluded. It has failed to finalize rules that require manufacturers to test priority chemicals that are already in use and is withdrawing proposed testing standards. It is relying instead on "voluntary" compliance by industry. It is retreating on protection against asbestos, a known dangerous substance.

Rejecting A Protective Cancer Policy. Long-term testing using laboratory animals is a scientifically sound way of identifying likely human carcinogens. The other generally accepted approach is through epidemiological studies comparing people exposed to a possible carcinogen with those who are not exposed.

Epidemiological studies are always costly, are usually relatively insensitive, and are often difficult or impossible to do. Many cancers do not show up until years after the exposure; most people are exposed to a great many carcinogens during their lives, which makes it hard to isolate the effect of one substance; and it is often difficult to find a suitable group of people who have not been exposed to particular substances, for comparison with others who have been. Animal tests, on the other hand, can be done under controlled conditions and can provide clearcut results. The International Agency for Research on Cancer, a federal interagency panel, and many other scientific groups have recommended that carcinogens identified in well-conducted animal tests be treated as potential human carcinogens. Up until now, government agencies have done so. A number of pesticides and carcinogens found in the workplace have been regulated on that basis.

President Reagan's EPA has suddenly reversed the established policy.

- Dr. John Todhunter, the new EPA Assistant Administrator for Toxics, decided that results of valid animal tests of formaldehyde, plus the fact of widespread human exposure, were not a sufficient basis for protective action. This decision flies in the face of the scientific consensus. It reverses EPA's former prudent approach of assessing and regulating cancer risks *before* they affect human beings.

Consulting Privately with Industry. In the fall of 1980 EPA received the results of animal experiments indicating that formaldehyde and di(2–ethylhexyl)phthalate (DEHP), both widely used chemicals, are carcinogens. Formaldehyde is used in plywood, particle board, home insulation, furniture, and fabrics, cosmetics, and toothpaste. DEHP is used in hundreds of plastic products, including building materials, food wrappers, toys, rubber baby pants, and milking machine hoses. After receiving the animal data, the staff of EPA recommended formal proceedings to determine the extent of the risk to human health, and action by EPA to limit human exposure.

Instead, the new leaders at EPA

- Convened a series of private meetings with industry—the Formaldehyde Institute, the Chemical Manufacturer's Association, Exxon, and others—to evaluate the studies and the risk of the substances.
- Did not notify or invite the public, environmentalists who had formally requested action on formaldehyde and DEHP, or even some of EPA's top cancer experts.
- After the meetings, rejected the prior staff recommendations and refused to institute proceedings (priority assessment) on the two chemicals.

Later, in a separate action, the Consumer Product Safety Commission concluded that the evidence against formaldehyde was compelling and banned urea formaldehyde foam insulation.

Relying on Voluntary Compliance by Industry. The Toxic Substances Control Act requires EPA to set rules for industry to test the safety of existing chemicals that a committee of experts concludes may pose a risk of cancer or injury to health or the environment. A 1981 court order requires EPA to issue test rules or explain why testing is unnecessary for 37 priority chemicals in the next two years. Instead of moving ahead with this critical task, EPA has

- Failed to issue pending test rules and delayed action on additional rules.
- Cut back sharply on resources necessary to develop test rules.
- Engaged in negotiations with industry to substitute "voluntary" testing for legal requirements.

Under another section of TSCA, the manufacturer of a new chemical must give EPA advance notice so that EPA can review the data available on potential hazards to human health. In 1982, EPA will receive 500 to 1000 such notices. EPA has:

- Failed to finalize the program for new chemical reporting.
- Cut back review staff, so that most notices of new chemical manufacture will receive only rubber-stamp review.
- Retreated from efforts to set minimum standards for data to be submitted by the manufacturers of new chemicals.
- Begun developing a rule at the request of the Chemical Manufacturers Association to exempt an estimated 75 percent of new chemicals from the notice requirement.

Retreating on Control of Known Dangerous Substances. Asbestos fibers cause asbestosis (fibrosis of the lungs), cancer of the lungs and digestive tract, and mesothelioma. Despite the proven health hazards of asbestos, the new EPA has

- Cut back on efforts to identify schools in which building materials expose children to asbestos.
- Weakened the warning on asbestos in schools approved by its own Science Advisory Committee.

At least 3 million students and 250,000 teachers may be affected by the retreat from protection against asbestos in schools.

Polychlorinated biphenyls (PCBs) are extremely toxic industrial chemicals. They have been widely used in electrical transformers, and they are pervasive in our environment. They are present in human breast milk and adipose tissue at toxicologically significant levels. PCB contamination has closed several rivers to fishing. In 1979 the leakage of 200 gallons of PCBs from a single transformer at the Pierce Packing Plant in Billings, Montana contaminated feed and food in 19 states and required the destruction of millions of dollars worth of contaminated livestock and food. Congress included in TSCA a provision that EPA ban the use of PCBs.

Under the Carter Administration, EPA issued regulations exempting the vast majority of PCBs in use from the ban. These regulations were overturned in court. Now, EPA is studying the question of new regulations, but has reduced the resources available to carry out the Congressional mandate.

Air Pollution

The Clean Air Act, our flagship environmental law, is under attack. The Reagan Administration's legislative proposals, regulatory changes, and budget actions are crippling the nation's clean air program. They threaten to bring back an era of dangerous, damaging, dirty air.

Preamble

Air pollution can kill people and make them ill; it attacks the natural environment; it destroys proper-

ty. Air pollution of various kinds causes or aggra-
vates cancer, emphysema, bronchitis, heart disease,
and other diseases. Acid rain destroys lakes and
forests. Ozone causes billions of dollars in crop
damage.

The clean air legislation passed a dozen years ago
and strengthened five years ago requires EPA, with
the help of the states, to clean up our air. For a
decade there was progress. A start has been made on
controlling pollution from automobiles, powerplants, smelters, refineries, and scores of other
sources.

But enormous tasks remain: ensuring that existing
nationwide health standards are met; regulating
highly toxic pollutants, such as benzene and arsenic,
that are still uncontrolled; controlling acid rain, and
inspecting existing controls to ensure that they continue to work.

Charges

Instead of tackling these tasks, the Administration
has marched backwards, abandoning the goal of
clean air.

Weakening National Clean Air Standards. The
Administration has proposed or supported amendments that would emasculate the Clean Air Act, has
dragged its feet on issuing regulations the law requires, and has abolished or watered down existing
regulations. Specifically, the Administration has
called for amendments to the law that would

- Weaken health standards to cover only so-called
  "significant risks." This means abandoning protection of specially sensitive groups such as children,
  the elderly, people with heart and lung disease, and
  others. The Congress has already blocked this
  attack on health standards.
- Allow deadlines for attaining the air quality standards that protect the public health to slip from 1982
  and 1987 to as late as 1993.
- Weaken auto emissions standards to allow more
  than a doubling of nitrogen oxide and carbon mon-

oxide emissions—a change that would expose millions of people in as many as 16 major urban areas to continued unhealthy air.

- Cripple the requirement that new cars must meet emission standards before they are sold and the provisions for recall when they do not.
- Do away with requirements that, in polluted areas, new sources of pollution (such as powerplants, refineries, chemical plants) use the most effective pollution controls available.
- Repeal protection for areas with air that is still clean, thus allowing new polluters to locate there and use less than the most effective pollution control technology.
- Drastically weaken the carrot-and-stick provisions by which the federal government encourages states to adopt effective pollution control plans. Conscientious states that adopt good plans would be at the mercy of industries which threaten to move to states having weaker controls.
- Allow greatly increased pollution of the air in National Parks and wilderness areas.

While mounting this assault on the law itself, EPA has taken administrative action to undo existing clean air requirements and has failed to issue long-overdue regulations. Some of these changes are subtle but far-reaching. For example, the Clean Air Act program to meet health standards in polluted areas depends on review by the states of proposals to build new industrial sources of pollution. Illegally redefining the word "source," EPA has effectively exempted most new polluting industrial installations from state reviews.

EPA has also

- Proposed to weaken by up to 5 times heavy truck emission standards, even though the National Commission on Air Quality found that emissions from heavy trucks must be controlled if we are to meet national health standards for air quality.
- Proposed to weaken the automobile emissions standard for hydrocarbons to permit an increase of approximately 25 percent in hydrocarbon emissions

(one of the constituents of photochemical smog).
- Proposed to weaken particulate emissions standards for diesel automobiles, the fastest growing and least controlled part of the automobile fleet.
- Failed to develop a particulate standard for diesel trucks.
- Failed to set required standards for industrial boilers and the most dangerous fine particulates.

The Administration has even proposed a retreat in control of lead, a pollutant which is especially dangerous to children. EPA itself has sponsored recent research which shows that even extremely low blood levels of lead affect the brain patterns of young children. Yet EPA has

- Developed proposals to allow increased use of lead in gasoline, thereby increasing human exposure, most significantly the exposure of inner city children. These proposals reverse a longstanding policy of the federal government to protect the health of the nation's children by rducing lead in the environment.

Failing to Act on Toxic Air Pollution. The Reagan Administraton's failure to move on toxic air pollution is especially threatening to millions of Americans who live in the shadow of chemical plants, coke ovens, and other factories which emit chemicals that can cause cancer and other deadly diseases. Recent research indicates that as much as 10 to 20 percent of lung cancer is due to air pollution. According to EPA, more than 300 plants in 39 states and territories emit large amounts of unregulated chemicals that are known or suspected to cause cancer or other serious diseases. Yet, after years of study, EPA has

- Failed to act on a list of 37 pollutants which threaten severe hazards to human health.
- Cut the budget for action on toxic air pollutants so sharply that it may be more than a decade before action on all these chemicals is even begun.

Failing to Act on Acid Rain. From West Virginia to

Maine, aquatic life in lakes and streams is dying. Thousands of lakes in Minnesota alone are in jeopardy, and hundreds are dead as sulfur from industrial stacks creates acid precipitation. In many states, acid rain is blamed for damaging forests and farmland and eroding buildings. Acid rain is a disaster that is real and growing.

The Reagan Administration claims that more study is needed before acting to control acid rain. The Administration opposes strengthening the Clean Air Act to mandate control measures. The Administration even seeks to weaken controls in current law limiting sulphur emissions from new plants. Even the words "acid rain" are out of fashion at EPA: Mrs. Gorsuch prefers the expression "non-buffered precipitation."

The Reagan Administration wants changes in the Clean Air Act to

- Exempt new large industrial coal-fired boilers from requirements that assure that a minimum percentage of sulfur oxides are removed from their emissions.
- Allow extensions of deadlines for meeting sulfur dioxide standards, which would allow delays and relaxations until 1993.

The Reagan Administration is also, by administrative action, changing the sulfur emission levels allowed from existing sources. It has

- Increased authorized sulfur dioxide emissions by 1.5 million tons a year, a very significant amount. Nationwide SO_2 emissions are currently 29 million tons per year.

The Administration has also undone a requirement proposed two years ago that powerplants with tall smoke stacks must reduce their SO_2 emissions by 412,000 tons per year. Now, EPA

- Is requiring a reduction of only 166,800 tons per year of SO_2 emissions from powerplants with tall stacks. Since present SO_2 emissions from tall stacks are over 500,000 tons per year, this means that more than 333,000 tons will still be contributing to acid rain in states and nations downwind of the powerplants.

Although the Reagan Administration has provided extra funds for acid rain research ($22 million for FY 1983, up $12 million over FY 1982), the addition may have a fatal drawback if research is simply being "accelerated" for a 5–year study, instead of the 10–year study originally planned by EPA. Many of the most serious effects of acid rain do not show up in the first 5 years.

Decreasing Enforcement. EPA has reduced the credibility and effectiveness of the entire regulatory program by a sudden and radical decrease in enforcement actions.

- After a series of jolting reorganizations and sharp budget cuts, the cases filed in federal court have declined almost 75 percent since Mrs. Gorsuch took office.
- Gorsuch personally undercut enforcement when she agreed in a private meeting with corporate officials to look the other way when Thriftway Refiners violated the Clean Air Act by increasing the amount of lead they put in their gasoline.

Reducing Research and Monitoring. Budget cuts proposed by the Reagan Administration will cripple research for air programs. Overall, the Reagan budget for FY 1983 proposes cuts of 23 percent from the level of two years ago in air quality. Specifically, the Reagan Administration budget would

- Eliminate human epidemiological research on the health effects of air pollution.
- Cut clinical research on health effects by 50 percent, eliminating investigation of volatile organic chemicals.
- Cut research on hazardous air pollutants severely. The Agency will look at three hazardous pollutants in 1983. At that rate, it will take a decade to examine the list of substances deemed priority because of their threat to human health.

The budget for monitoring air programs and assisting states has also been drastically cut. The proposed Reagan budget for FY 1983 would

- Cut back by 40 percent monitoring of air quality to determine the levels and kinds of pollution already present in our air.
- Cut grants and technical assistance to state air programs by 30 percent, thus crippling state efforts to implement clean air requirements.

An unprecedented Congressional hearing was held in July 1982 on "EPA oversight" by five House subcommittees— Energy and Natural Resources; Investigations and Oversight; Natural Resources, Agricultural Research and the Environment; Health and the Environment; Commerce, Transportation and Tourism.

Testimony at that hearing included that of Russell W. Peterson, president of the National Audubon Society:

We are all appalled at the spectacle of EPA, entrusted with protecting our nation's health and environment, consciously abdicating that responsibility, and at times even seeming to play the role of chief spokesman for polluters.

Peterson, former Republican governor of Delaware and former chairman of the Council of Environmental Quality under Presidents Nixon and Ford, declared:

Contrary to the Reagan ideology, environmental protection is good for the economy. It has created many more jobs than it has displaced. A whole new pollution-control industry has come into being.

The economy has not been "burdened" by antipollution efforts: health protection results alone (to say nothing of preserving and enhancing quality of life) have more than repaid our pollution control expenditures. In other words, the premise on which they base their anti-environment campaign is wrong. Where are their facts to show that environmental regulations hurt our economy? To profess that something is so doesn't make it so. But admittedly when people on high conduct a campaign to tell it like it isn't, many will believe them.

We ask you to reject the administration's anti-environmental policy and redirect EPA to function as the public intended, and Congress mandated, and its name indicates—that is to say, as our Environmental Protection Agency.

As Gaylord Nelson, chairman of the Wilderness Society, testified:

Tragically, at this precise moment in history when the circumstances demand not just a continuation of past constructive policies, but a vigorous expansion of our address to the whole spectrum of resource issues, we have an Administration that is turning the clock back because it is either blind to the problem and ignorant of the consequences or recklessly prepared to dissipate the resources of future generations for short-term political gain and illusory economic benefits.

We are witnessing a wholesale dismantling of the environmental achievements and gains of the past decade and a half. It is being done by a series of executive and administrative actions without review by Congress and beyond the view of the public. Their techniques and tactics involve non-enforcement, weak enforcement or perverse enforcement of the law by administrators and lawyers who were appointed for the specific purpose of frustrating the will of Congress and the vast majority of the people as repeatedly expressed through public opinion polls.

Nelson, a former Senator, spoke of how "by massive budget cuts they have seriously crippled the Environmental Protection Agency, and their proposed budget for next year will effectively destroy its capacity to administer and enforce the major responsibilities within its jurisdiction."

He examined, among other things, the situation concerning the EPA and pesticides:

EPA has identified 520 active pesticide ingredients. Only 20 were evaluated in the last two years; 500 more ingredients remain plus any new ones that may be developed. The Administration budget proposes to evaluate 15 more ingredients in FY 83—more than the Agency has ever evaluated in a single year—while cutting resources in half from FY 81 levels. Even assuming that EPA successfully completes its evaluations at this rate, *the remaining active chemical ingredients will not be evaluated until the year 2017*, not counting any new chemicals that are developed. These substances are intentional poisons applied directly to what we eat. They also contaminate both our land and water.

Merilyn B. Reeves, a vice president of the League of Women Voters of the United States, testified:

It is our observation that under the guise of "regulatory reform" and the President's economic recovery program, opportunities for providing for public information and consultation are being stifled. In their place, EPA has instituted the ostrich policy. Rather than facing up to our nation's serious environmental problems, this Administration would prefer to bury its head in the sand.

Margaret Tileston of the Sierra Club spoke of how "EPA's enforcement record over the past year has been dreadful" and of toxic chemicals:

Over 40,000 chemical products are in commerce in the United States. Six hundred to a thousand new products will come to EPA next year for premanufacture review. We have little information on what the vast majority of these products do to living organisms, how they enter our environment, how they travel through it, where they may be accumulating, or how many people are exposed to them. Congress passed the Toxic Substances Control Act in 1976 to require EPA to screen new and existing chemicals and to protect the public from those that endanger human health. The proposed FY 1983 budget would slow that process to a crawl, so that it will be decades before we even learn what is dangerous. By then it will be too late for many Americans.

And Senator Patrick J. Leahy of Vermont told the hearing how "the threat to public health of the administration's policies is unique," that the Reagan administration "has undertaken an unprecedented assault on our institutional capability to control pollution."

He chronicled a sequence of EPA "mismanagement."

1. Ms. Gorsuch abolished the enforcement division on July 1, 1981, in spite of the fact that a major consultant's report warned her that the "case for making that change now does not overcome the costs of the disruption a reorganization would cause" and that such a reorganization "can be highly damaging to staff morale, productivity, and to an office's key programs."

2. Between July 1981 and May 1982, the enforcement division went through a major reorganization every eleven weeks.

3. For six of the last thirteen months, there was no overall legal director for the Environmental Protection Agency with the result that the two deputies were continually feuding over control of policy.

4. Enforcement policies were so confused that ten months after the first reorganization and four months after the second reorganization, EPA's chief financial officer still had to ask Administrator Gorsuch to decide the basic issue of "what functions should (the Office of Legal and Enforcement Counsel) manage."

5. Management controls and policies were so weak in the critical hazardous waste area that one regional office with severe hazardous waste problems delegated all inspection to the states while another region with relatively few problems led the nation in inspections.

6. Because of mismanagement, for six out of the last thirteen months, there were only about ten attorneys in the enforcement section of the Office of Legal and Enforcement Counsel.

7. As a result of the mismanagement of EPA's enforcement division, by any objective measure, enforcement efforts have dropped by 70–80%.

Leahy declared:

> The American people want environmental protection. They want their health and their children's health protected. They want clean air to breathe and clean water to drink. Indeed, a recent Roper poll found that 70% of the public want EPA to be as tough or tougher than it was in the past.
>
> The American people want an environmental policy that works. It is time they had it.

As Representative James Scheuer, the chairman of one subcommittee, phrased it: "The Environmental Protection Agency has been on the cutting edge of the administration's inglorious retreat across the spectrum of environmental protection."

Representative James Florio, chairman of another subcommittee which took part in the hearing, said, "Over the last year and a half we have witnessed nothing less than a fundamental, radical attempt to reverse a decade of environmental progress." The Environmental Protection Agency "has effectively dropped the 'Protection' from its name."

Horror Story Sampler

The horror stories about how the earth and life on it are being poisoned for private profit with official approval are abundant and tragic and cry out for the madness to be stopped.

***

Formaldehyde, it has finally been realized, is a deadly chemical. Developed by German chemist August Wilhelm von Hofmann in 1867, its applications in the more than a century that followed have become widescale: it's used as an embalming fluid, as a component of toothpaste, in shampoos, in cosmetics, as a fertilizer additive, in plywood, in paints, it's the stuff that keeps paper towels bonded and maintains the "press" in permanent-press fabrics.

In the 1970's, urea-formaldehyde, some 16 million gallons of it—a material with shaving cream-like texture whipped up from formaldehyde resin—was pumped into the walls of a half-million homes in America for insulation.

The health problems that caused led to a product investigation, done as is usually the case by the makers of the substance. The Chemical Industry Institute of Toxicology, a facility in North Carolina funded by U.S. chemical companies, began a study of formaldehyde in 1978. The following year it reported that the inhalation of but 15 parts per million of formaldehyde in air caused nasal tumors in 40% of the test animals exposed.

The formaldehyde industry, which annually produces six

billion pounds of the stuff and sells it for $300 million, insisted as is often the pattern that the animal-cancer connection didn't mean that formaldehyde is cancer-causing to humans, too.

A panel of 17 scientists from seven different federal agencies disagreed and in 1980, based on the findings of the Chemical Industry Institute study and further research at New York University, ruled that formaldehyde "poses a cancer risk to humans."

EPA scientists then began drafting regulations to govern formaldehyde.

On her first day on the job, May 20, 1981, the new EPA administrator, Anne Gorsuch, had a letter waiting from S. John Byington, a lobbyist for the Formaldehyde Institute, which declared: "We realize as we write this that you have been formally in the job for only a couple of hours, but the movement of the bureaucracy waits for no person."

What then followed was a series of meetings between representatives of the Formaldehyde Institute, other industry representatives, and EPA officials at which formaldehyde and any proposed restrictions on it were discussed.

A principal in those discussions was Dr. John Todhunter who Mrs. Gorsuch named her assistant administrator for pesticides and toxic substances and who previously had represented opponents of pesticide regulations and had been "scientific advisor" of the industry-funded American Council on Science and Health.

The American Council on Science and Health lists the same telephone and mailing address as the Washington lobbying office of Byington of the Formaldehyde Institute.

In the end, the EPA reversed itself on formaldehyde with one career EPA scientist, Richard Dailey, resigning as a result, as a matter of conscience.

Now formaldehyde is no longer among the chemicals that the EPA considers a possible toxic substance under the Toxic Substances Control Act.

At one point, Todhunter wrote a memo urging that formaldehyde not be put under regulation despite a "limited but suggestive epidemiological base" that "human problems with formaldehyde carcinogenicity may be of low incidence."

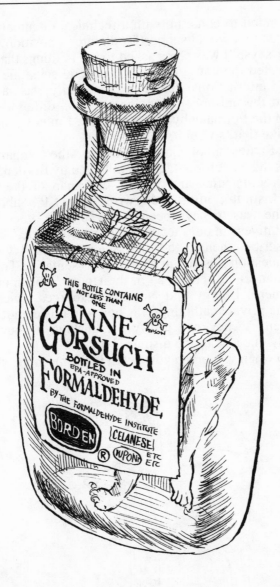

And EPA scientists wrote a memo which declared that "Waiting, in essence, 'till the bodies fall' before taking action may afford inadequate protection of the public."

Dailey resigned from the EPA after he and other scientists

were directed to come up with a technical document on formaldehyde that would support Todhunter's position.

Dailey says: "I was being asked to put in things that I didn't feel reflected the consensus of the general scientific community. The international scientific community was saying one thing and the only people saying anything different was the EPA and the Formaldehyde Institute . . . I'm not going to live my life like that, so I quit."

James Ramey, an official of Celanese—the company which produces the most formaldehyde followed by Borden, Dupont and Georgia-Pacific—and who is chairman of the Formaldehyde Institute, afterwards wrote the EPA about how pleased he was to have been involved with other industry representatives "in our meetings on formaldehyde."

He described them as the "first Science Court."

"The question raised," declared Representative Toby Moffett of Connecticut, chairman of the House Subcommittee on Environment, Energy and Natural Resources which investigated the private gatherings, "is how—in this democracy—a government agency can justify establishing a court which hears only one side of the dispute."

And so when you brush your teeth in the morning, shampoo

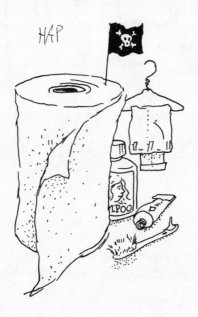

your hair, hold a paper towel—just put on your shirt and pants—you will likely be exposed to a cancer-causing substance.

***

People are constantly being exposed to poisons through cosmetics which commonly are composed, in part, of toxins. Here, too, the public is not being protected.

"We want to believe that the federal government vigilantly protects the public from any abuses or negligence in the cosmetic industry. But Washington is rapidly losing what feeble regulatory powers it once wielded in this field," noted the Science Action Coalition of Washington in its *Consumer's Guide to Cosmetics.*

The book was published in 1980 following a cut in the staff of the cosmetics division of the FDA—from 81 in 1979 to 45— and a chopping of the budget from $3 million to $2 million.

"It is sobering to realize," declared Science Action Coalition, "that industry is spending almost a billion dollars a year to promote its products—roughly 500 times" the government budget for public protection.

Further, although cosmetics are ostensibly "covered" under federal food and drug legislation they—unlike food and drugs—don't even require a showing by their manufacturers that they are safe.

Noted the Science Action Coalition: "Even if the FDA had enforcement powers, it wouldn't even know whom to regulate! It has registered only 825 of an estimated 2,000-3,000 cosmetic manufacturers."

And the poisons that cosmetics are loaded with range from a classic poison, lye, used in hair straighteners, to cancer-causing nitrosamines in shampoos and skin creams, and another carcinogen—2,4-diaminoanisole (2,4DAA)—a standard ingredient in hair dyes.

Stressed *Consumer's Guide to Cosmetics:* "The FDA has compiled a preliminary list of about 100 compounds used in cosmetics that are suspected carcinogens or teratogens." But "very little is known about the long-term toxicity of many of the 8,000 beauty aids now in the marketplace, since few have been tested adequately."

***

Once, a hunter could bag wild ducks and geese and have the purest of foods. Not any more. On the West Coast, endrin—a pesticide up to 300 times more toxic than DDT for some species—has contaminated wildfowl; on the East Coast wildfowl have become poisoned with PCB's.

The Montana Department of Health in 1981 recommended unsuccessfully that the waterfowl hunting season be cancelled in Montana and 17 other Western states because of high levels of endrin found in ducks and geese on the Pacific and Central flyways.

The cause was endrin sprayed on wheat fields in Montana, Wyoming, South Dakota and Colorado.

Endrin has a long history of chemical destruction. In the early 1960's, kills of many millions of fish in the Mississippi River were connected to a series of endrin discharges from a Velsicol Chemical Corporation plant producing endrin in Memphis, Tennessee. The EPA then cancelled some uses of endrin (on tobacco and ornaments) but balked at attempts to have the pesticide banned. In the 1970's, the spraying of endrin on 5.5 million acres of farmland in Kansas and Oklahoma led to widescale deaths of livestock, wildlife and domestic animals.

Also in the 1970's, endrin was determined to have been the cause of the poisoning of many people in Qatar in the Persian Gulf who had eaten bread made from flour contaminated with endrin. Seven hundred persons required hospitalization; 24 died.

A quarter of an ounce of endrin can kill in less than an hour. It is a carcinogen. It can lead to birth defects. Small amounts can cause severe nausea, convulsions and damage to the brain and nervous system.

A single serving of a duck contaminated with the concentrations of endrin found in wildfowl in the West in 1981 could poison a child, authorities warned.

"The birds should not be consumed," said Montana Health Commissioner John Drynan. He voiced fears about pregnant women having "deformed" children if they ate endrin-contaminated wildfowl.

"The ramifications of this spraying are mind-boggling," said Dr. Drynan. "One of the things I am concerned about is the leaching process. If we wait a year or two, will endrin end up in our ground water supplies and well water?"

Indeed, endrin remains a hazard in the environment for at least a dozen years after being applied. Its label advises farmers to keep livestock off sprayed fields for a year. Endrin passes up the food chain and lodges in fat tissue of birds, animals and people, remaining for years.

Testing for Montana at Rai-Tech labs in Madison, Wisconsin in 1982 showed that concentrations of endrin in wildfowl sampled were as high as 2.98 parts per million—*ten times* the .03 per million federal allowable limit for domestic poultry. And the testing found not only endrin in high concentrations but 18 other toxic pesticides in the wildfowl sampled, too.

But the EPA declared that the endrin levels in Western wildfowl was not a danger because federal levels are established with a wide leeway, EPA officials ruled.

Montana Governor Ted Schwinden created a Pesticide Advisory Council to examine the situation. Its members include the distributor of much of the endrin used in the West, and an aerial pesticide sprayer who stresses, "We haven't really established there is an endrin problem."

Meanwhile, warnings have been issued for people not to eat too many wild ducks or geese in the West, and to cut out the fatty tissue of wildfowl to reduce the amount of pesticide that would be ingested.

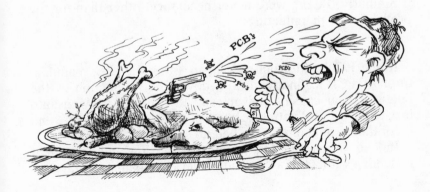

This type of warning has also recently been posted in the East where PCB's contaminate wildfowl.

A sample warning:

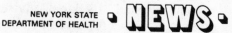

NEW YORK STATE
DEPARTMENT OF HEALTH

for release:
Wednesday, October 7, 1981

CONTACT: BARBARA THOMAS-NOBLE, DIRECTOR, PUBLIC AFFAIRS (518) 474-7354

DAVID AXELROD, M.D.
Commissioner

Albany, October 7 -- State Health Commissioner David Axelrod and

Environmental Conservation Commissioner Robert Flacke today recommended that,

on the basis of new information on the presence of PCBs in wild waterfowl,

certain precautions be taken before eating these game birds.

● Discard the skin and remove all visible fat before cooking. Contaminants tend to accumulate in fatty tissue; removal of fat will significantly reduce any contaminants present in the fowl.

● If the birds are stuffed, discard the stuffing since it will absorb the oils which contain the contaminants.

● Avoid consumption of merganser ducks. Contaminant levels in this species were greater than in the other species tested.

● Limit ingestion to two meals per month.

Other than for the profits of its manufacturers, endrin is not needed for wheat—less than 10% of U.S. wheat is treated with pesticides. Wheat is largely pest-resistent and what occasional damage cutworms, which endrin is supposed to kill, do is far less damage than endrin causes.

Similarly, PCB's were never necessary, other than for the profit of their manufacturer.

***

In the 1970's, Monsanto Company, the sole U.S. manufacturer of PCB's, finally slowed down the production of the potent cancer-causing poison, and then ended it. Monsanto insisted it was not acting because of government pressure and it continued to claim PCB's had no substitute.

Indeed, our would-be protectors were slow and delinquent in dealing with a toxin that had earlier been banned in Japan—

and which Japan was able to do quite well without.

Monsanto began churning out PCB's—the acronym for polychlorinated biphenyls—in 1929. It produced mammoth quantities of the poison which researchers have been unable to find a safe level for: doses as low as one-half part per million and even 25 parts per billion have had carcinogenic and mutagenic effects.

Monsanto produced up to *85 million pounds* of PCB's *each year,* a total of 1.5 billion pounds of the stuff. It has had a wide array of uses: for carbonless paper, in paint, in inks, in adhesives, in plastics, in caulking, in Xerox toner, and especially as an insulating fluid in electrical components such as capacitators and transformers.

Now, virtually all Americans are estimated to carry some amount of PCB's in their systems. A survey by the EPA in 1979 put the figure for the average American at two parts per million.

An EPA study in 1975–1976 found PCB's in virtually all the samples tested of mothers' milk—up to ten times the maximum daily intake level set by the FDA. "Indeed, if human milk were marketed in interstate commerce, much of it would be seized and condemned by the FDA" as a result of PCB's pollution, noted the 1979 book, *Malignant Neglect* by the Environmental Defense Fund and Robert H. Boyle.

Besides being in wildfowl, PCB's have become ubiquitous in other forms of life. They're in 90.2% of freshwater fish in the United States according to a 1974 survey by the U.S. Fish and Wildlife Service. They've been found in amounts as high as 340 parts per million in fish taken downstream from two General Electric plants along the Hudson River in New York State which long dumped PCB's—at one point with an EPA permit to dump the poison into the river. PCB's are in animals worldwide, including even Arctic polar bears where they've been found at levels up to eight parts per million.

"It seems safe to conclude that PCB's are present in varying concentrations in every species of wildlife on earth," says Dr. George Harvey of the Woods Hole Oceanographic Institution.

The toxic qualities of PCB's were known for years. In the 1930's, Monsanto workers involved with PCB's manufacture began developing disfiguring skin eruptions of chloracne. In 1943, the New York State Department of Labor published a report connecting chloracne, dermatitis and deaths from liver damage among workers handling equipment containing PCB's and closely-related chemicals to this exposure.

"Thus, both Monsanto and the government were aware of the extremely dangerous nature of these chemicals four or five decades go, but nothing was done to restrict their use until the late 1970's," wrote Lewis Regenstein in *America the Poisoned*. "Both industry and government forfeited an opportunity to prevent our present environmental crisis with PCB's, at untold cost in lives lost, people's health ruined, and the environment poisoned." Some forty years—and 1.5 billion pounds of PCB's—later, our country is faced with a toxic chemical contamination problem of immense proportions that may, in the end, prove insoluble."

The production of PCB's was banned in Japan after a 1968 incident in which a thousand residents on the Japanese island of Kyusha ate rice oil which had become contaminated with PCB's. Ten people soon died and the remainder developed what became known as *yusho* (rice oil) disease. Symptoms included loss of hair, discharges from the eyes, jaundice, dizziness, nausea, impotence and other sexual disorders, numbness, darkening of the skin, loss of vision. There was subsequently an abnormally high rate of cancer deaths among the "yusho" victims. And there were birth defects among infants born to women who had ingested the PCB's-polluted rice oil.

Korishi Saito, in charge of supervision of Japan's chemical industry in the Ministry of International Trade and Industry at the time, says his nation had no trouble ending production of PCB's in 1972 and putting substitutes into use.

"Judging from our experience with PCB's, it is obvious that we have to be careful in introducing new chemical substances into commercial usage," he declares.

Meanwhile, in America, supposed government protectors were doing little or nothing. And Monsanto was maintaining that nothing could substitute for its PCB's.

As this 1970 Monsanto statement phrased it:

NEWS

Monsanto

E. V. John
(314) 694-2891
PUBLIC RELATIONS DEPARTMENT
Monsanto Company
800 N. Lindbergh Boulevard
St. Louis, Missouri 63166

FOR RELEASE   IMMEDIATELY 1970

MONSANTO CITES
ACTIONS TAKEN ON
ENVIRONMENTAL ISSUE

ST. LOUIS, July 16 -- Monsanto Company, sole U.S.
producer of an industrial chemical called polychlorinated biphenyl
(PCB), today said recent political charges and sensational
headlines about the chemical causing "a major ecological
crisis" completely ignore voluntary actions the company has
taken to restrict use of the material.

"PCB is used in electrical equipment as a safety
fluid. It has replaced combustible oil products which have,
on many occasions, exploded and burned, causing deaths and
injury to human life. Today state and local laws all over the
country require the use of non-flammable fluids in certain
electrical equipment as a safety feature. At the moment, there
are no substitutes available which equal the safety performance
of PCB."

The company said it would cease producing PCB's for some
uses but not, it stressed, because Monsanto had "been pressured into action by any legislation or organized group."

And, it said it would continue to make over 25 million
pounds a year of PCB's for "'closed-system' uses such as
electrical components and heat-transfer systems."

With the passage of the Toxic Substances Control Act in 1976 and continued global uproar over PCB's, the company in that year issued a reported entitled: "Polychlorinated Biphenyls, A Risk/Benefit Dilemma" which spoke of the disruption that would be caused if PCB's were no longer produced and of the "irreplaceable role" PCB's "have played in electrical and industrial applications for the past 45 years."

Japan, a highly-industrialized nation, had found substitutes for PCB's but purportedly America could not!

In 1977, the EPA issued restricted new uses of PCB's leaving a massive hole when it granted "hardship exemptions" to virtually all who made pre-existing use of them. The Environmental Defense Fund brought a lawsuit against the EPA for the blanket exemptions. In 1979, the EPA finally got around to banning the production of PCB's, and also set weak disposal standards for the estimated 758 million pounds of PCB's still in use.

Federal regulatory agencies have been "asleep" on PCB's, said *Malignant Neglect,* and "needlessly delayed action."

The EPA continues to stall on PCB's. In August 1982, because of federal court orders imposed on it, the EPA said it would bar—in 1985—transformers containing PCB's from areas where food could be contaminated. The agency refused to order removal of the large majority of transformers containing PCB's that would still remain. The Environmental Defense Fund noted that transformers leak 25,000 pounds of PCB's into the environment annually but the EPA said the replacement of all transformers would cost industry too much money. And the EPA, under the same court orders, announced it would—in 1988—require the replacement of 1.5 million capacitors containing PCB's used by utilities. Capacitors are estimated to leak 439,000 pounds of PCB's a year.

An example of the governmental attitude toward PCB's-pollution came when a fire and explosion in a New York State government office building in Binghamton in 1981 caused PCB's to spew from a transformer into the building's ventilation system.

State officials minimized the incident; 500 people were exposed to toxins before the state closed the building.

Then New York Governor Hugh Carey went to the structure and announced he would "drink a glass of PCB's." Lucky for him he never did. The 18-story building is still closed. Signs posted on it read: "CONTAMINATED."

"I used to be a true believer in the state," says Lois Whittemore who was a guard at the building when the explosion occurred. She fears that the PCB's she absorbed will cause injury to her or a child she might bear. "I thought they knew what the hell they were doing. But now my philosophy is if it makes sense and it is totally logical, the state won't buy it."

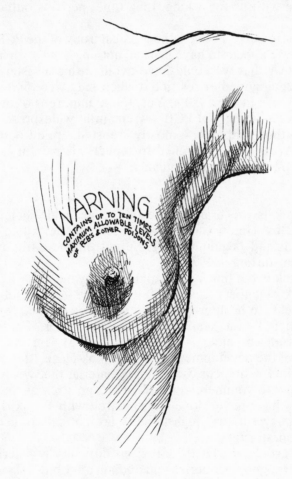

In addition to the many hundreds of millions of pounds of PCB's still in use or already dispersed into the environment, the EPA estimates that some 150 million pounds of the poison lie buried in landfills across America—much of it encased inside metal transformers and capacitors, "closed-systems," which as they rust and corrode are ceasing from being closed with the PCB's oozing out.

"Despite the government's unwillingness to face up to the PCB problem," wrote Regenstein in *America the Poisoned*, "it cannot be ignored; it will not go away. These chemicals will be with us for a long, long time, perhaps outlasting our society."

He stressed: "Perhaps the greatest irony of the PCB tragedy is that we appear to have learned nothing from it. In hindsight, it is clear that we could have avoided this disaster if PCB's had been banned or restricted when they were first shown to be so toxic in the 1930's. Yet, today hundreds of other toxic chemicals—potential PCB's—remain in widespread use, and over a thousand others, mostly untested, are introduced each year. We seem determined to repeat this painful experience with dozens of other chemicals."

***

Temik is the brand name of the pesticide aldicarb, concocted by Union Carbide and used on the potato fields of Long Island beginning in 1975 and on the citrus groves of Florida starting in 1978.

Temik is ten times more toxic than cyanide.

EPA scientists described it as "the most acutely toxic chemical" to be approved for registration by the agency.

"When I first heard of Temik," says Dr. Frederick W. Plapp, an entemologist at Texas A & M University where some of the development of Temik took place, "I thought of it as an interesting curiosity, not a material that would eventually go into commercial use." Dr. Plapp stresses that, "I personally have never done any research with Temik. I feel that materials with such high toxicity are not safe to use even in the laboratory."

Nevertheless, the EPA had no difficulty registering it for use throughout America—including on Long Island and in

Florida where the soil is sandy and relatively sterile.

Temik, which requires biological decay to break down, might persist in such soil, the Technical Advisory Committee of the Long Island Regional Planning Board and the Cooperative Extension Association of Suffolk County warned.

And, in fact, Temik failed to break down in such soil.

On Long Island, where 100,000 pounds of Temik were spread on potato fields each year from 1975 to 1980 when Union Carbide pulled it off the Long Island market, it has contaminated wells throughout the island's eastern portion. Amounts as high as 515 parts per billion, *74 times* the New York State limit for Temik of seven parts per billion, have been found. The Temik pollution was still giving no indication of a let-up on Long Island in 1982 and the Suffolk Department of Health Services was announcing that the poison "can be expected to remain" in the water table for 100 more years.

In Florida, where in 1981 a pesticide applicator died from exposure to Temik despite his wearing of protective gear, Temik has become an ingredient in many oranges.

The federal limit of 300 parts of Temik per billion in oranges—set that high, says the EPA, because people drink less orange juice than water—has even been found to be exceeded.

After newspaper and television reports about Temik contamination in the Florida citrus industry, Florida Governor Robert Graham in 1982 ordered tests for the chemical.

"They don't monitor pesticides on a regular basis at all," comments Victoria Churchill, an *Orlando Sentinel* reporter who wrote a story about Temik.

On Long Island, too, monitoring of Temik by local and state authorities was dismal. Reports in the local media and demands by environmentalists and others concerned about water purity finally triggered action. At one press conference, Dr. Martin Shepard declared that "it is not a question of chemicals or starvation. It's a matter of choosing farming methods in harmony with nature instead of insulting nature." Suffolk Legislator Wayne Prospect charged that he was "disgusted" with the State Department of Environmental Conservation and the Suffolk health department. "We have to look outside the government bureaucracies for help. I don't know who the bureaucracies are serving but it is not the people. A main function of government is to preserve the public health of its citizens. It's failing miserably."

Later, Charles Frommer, who when Temik was introduced on Long Island was director of the New York State Department of Environmental Conservation's Bureau of Pesticide Control, said, "It has all come as quite a surprise to us." Frommer had left the government by then to become director of regulatory affairs for the Velsicol Chemical Company.

A special subcommittee of the Suffolk County Legislature issued a report declaring:

> The EPA failed in its regulatory function by certifying Temik for use on Long Island farms. If in no other way, this failure can be identified by EPA's acceptance of research techniques, and conclusions, which Carbide itself has since termed inadequate. It is for this very reason that Suffolk County cannot rely upon EPA to prevent a recurrence of Temik's drastic scenario. Nor can the people look to EPA to assist in correcting a tragedy which EPA fostered. Guilt is but one of the many unfortunate relationships which EPA and the chemical companies share. EPA staff scientists often advance their careers by joining the ranks of the chemical corporations' employees. Moreover, corporate giants like Carbide perform the kind of research which EPA could not hope to duplicate. Consequently, there persists an unhealthy reliance by EPA upon Carbide. Temik's unfortunate history attests to this.

A Long Island chapter of Science for the People charged "bureaucratic mismanagement, needless public health risk and inadequate monitoring and analysis" by those in government who were supposed to be responsible for passing on and monitoring Temik.

Meanwhile, the toxic Temik remains in the water of eastern Long Island which relies solely on an underground water supply—like much of Florida—for its supply of potable water.

People on Long Island with Temik-contaminated water have been getting this letter from Union Carbide offering a water filter:

AGRICULTURAL PRODUCTS COMPANY, Inc.
270 PARK AVENUE, NEW YORK, N.Y. 10017

June 30, 1980

Union Carbide Agricultural Products Company, Inc. has been informed by the Suffolk County Department of Health Services that a test of your well water indicates a level of TEMIK® residue in excess of the New York State guideline of 7 parts per billion of aldicarb. The purpose of this letter is to offer those homeowners whose well water exceeds this independently established state guideline an installed water filtration system for their residence. This activated carbon filtration system has been successfully demonstrated, under actual Suffolk County conditions, to reduce aldicarb residues in well water to the guideline level of 7 parts per billion or less.

While detected residues have resulted in no adverse health effects, Union Carbide is providing these filtration systems free of charge as an extension of our effort, in cooperation with the Suffolk County Department of Health Services, to eliminate any concern that anyone may have with respect to trace levels of TEMIK® residues found in their water.

To request the installation of a filtration system, simply complete the attached order form, and mail it to Union Carbide Agricultural Products Company, Inc. in the enclosed envelope. Our representative will contact you within two (2) weeks of the receipt of your signed order form to make an appointment for the installation. This offer will remain available to you until August 29, 1980.

W. K. Stamer
Program Manager

Serious questions have been raised about the effectiveness of the filter. And Union Carbide, although initially providing a filter, refuses to supply costly filter elements replacements. It also refuses to provide Long Island officials data on Temik—claiming all such research is a "trade secret."

Health impacts of Temik contamination have begun to appear on Long Island. In 1982, Suffolk County issued findings of research showing a high incidence of miscarriages and neurologicial disorders among people with Temik in their water.

Union Carbide first reacted to the Temik contamination on Long Island by aggressively lobbying for an increase in the state limit of seven parts per billion. That didn't work amidst the public outrage although some politicians supported the idea.

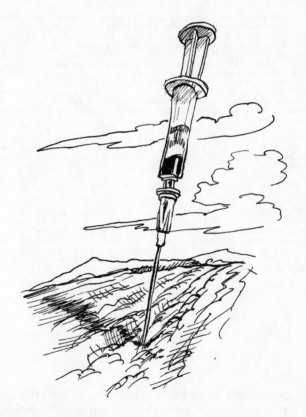

Later, the company took to pointing the finger of responsibility for Temik pollution to the EPA. "EPA is the governing body," declared R. L. Bertwell, product development manager for Temik for Union Carbide, at a public meeting on Temik pollution in 1982. "Don't single out me or Union Carbide." Someone spoke of a "revolving door" between chemical companies and regulatory agencies, of the two being best friends." Bertwell insisted that government bureaucrats are not "in our pocket, they in ours." He said it is "not all hugs and kisses . . . They're not in our camp."

The people at the hearing with poison in their wells didn't believe the man from Union Carbide.

***

"Are the materials you are working with slowly killing you?" asked Dr. Michael McCann at the start of a booklet directed not at chemical industry workers but artists and others who use arts and crafts materials.

"The range of dangerous materials is very broad," he continued in the *Health Hazards Manual For Artists*. "It includes traditional art materials like lead paints and pottery glazes, solvents, inks, welding fumes, wood and plastic dusts from sanding, and a wide variety of new plastics materials."

At the Manhattan office of the Center for Occupational Hazards, of which he is the director, McCann is commenting on U.S. government activity concerning poisons in art materials: "I don't think they've done a thing." Under the Reagan administration "there is a whole climate against regulation" and things weren't much better under Carter, he says.

The number of people involved in arts and crafts in America—and exposed to the many poisons in art materials—is immense, he stresses. There are between a half-million to a million professionals involved in arts in the U.S., says McCann, including an estimated 129,000 painters and sculptors, 100,000 commercial artists, 250,000 to 350,000 craftspeople and 70,000 to 80,000 art specialists in schools. He cites a Harris poll which found that 39% of the U.S. population over 16 are engaged in weaving, pottery, ceramics and woodworking and 16% involved in drawing, painting or sculpture and calculates the hobbyists in arts and crafts numbering between 75 and 80 million.

Then there are children,"almost all" of whom use arts and crafts material. "We're dealing with a vast number of people," says McCann.

All face exposure to poisons.

These include, he notes:

• Solvents like benzene, toluene, methylene chloride, n-hexane and perchloroethylene in lacquer and other thinners, paint removers, cleaners, aerosol sprays and plastics resins.

• Metals like lead, cadmium, manganese, chromium and uranium in pigments, pottery glazes, solders, photochemicals and alloys.

• Mineral dusts like crystalline silica and asbestos in stones, clays, pottery glazes, foundry sands, talcs and plastics fillers.

• Gases like chlorine, ozone, nitrogen dioxide and sulfur dioxide generated as a by-product of welding, photo-processes, acid etching, kiln and foundry firings and plastics decomposition.

• Other hazardous chemicals such as benzidine congener dyes, acids and alkalis used in arts and craft processes.

The Center for Occupational Hazards offers a course on art hazards and puts out a monthly, *Art Hazards Newsletter*.

It has been working in conjunction with the National Cancer Institute on a study to assess the "occupational health problems in the arts."

Preliminary results, says McCann, show that male artists have "significantly higher" rates of cancer of the brain, kidney and bladder and leukemia than the general population, and cancers of the colon, rectum and prostate are also "higher than expected." Women artists have been found to have "significantly higher" rates of cancer of the breast, lung and rectum than the general population.

This corroborates with the findings of studies involving deaths among professionals involved in arts conducted in Washington State, in England, Wales and in Japan, he continues.

What can be done?

Says McCann:

"First, some art materials should be reformulated to eliminate extremely toxic chemicals for which adequate substitutes exist. Examples include cadmium in silver solders, n-hexane in rubber cement thinners and other products, asbestos in talc and insulating materials, lead in enamels and pottery materials, benzidine congener dyes, etc. Adequate substitutes exist for all.

"Second, arts and crafts products need to be more adequately labeled with their contents, hazards, precautions, disposal. At present most art materials are not adequately labeled. The Federal Hazardous Substances Act only requires labeling for acute or immediate hazards, whereas many of the hazards faced by artists are chronic hazards. And even this law is not being obeyed in many instances.

"Third, and probably most important, artists, craftspeople, art teachers and students, hobbyists and children have to be educated about the hazards of their arts and crafts materials and how to work with them safely. One of the most important areas for this to occur is in the public schools and art schools. Unfortunately, at present most art teachers themselves do not have this training."

"CHILDREN BEWARE: Art Supplies In The Classroom" was a report done by the Joint New York State Assembly Standing Committee on Consumer Affairs and Protection released in June 1982. It involved a survey of 15 New York State school systems in which, it was found, children between kindergarten to the 12th grade were using art materials containing thirteen known or suspected carcinogens, two known or suspected mutagens (chemicals which can produce cell mutations), and eight known or suspected teratogens (chemicals capable of producing birth defects).

Some sixteen types of art materials were "found to be insufficiently labeled" with "information on potentially toxic ingredients and their possible health effects either inadequately detailed or nonexistent on product labels."

Emphasized the report, "Toxic chemicals are in common use in New York State schools."

The Assembly committee complained that manufacturers of art supplies "often" provided it with "inaccurate and unreliable sources of data, differing greatly from accepted medical and scientific sources" when it made inquiry about "various chemicals' health hazards." And, some 40% of the manufacturers didn't even reply to inquiries.

Said the report:

> Another aspect of this problem is that children, particularly young children, may misuse art materials. Young children have a well-known tendency to put things in their mouths or they may deliberately inhale art materials in order to achieve "glue-sniffer's high". Often, the ingestion of hazardous materials is unintentional, as when children fail to wash paint off their hands and eat, drink, or bite their fingernails.
>
> Parents, teachers or public health officials who become aware of this problem and try to safeguard children by eliminating entirely or reducing to a minimum the number of toxic art supplies quickly confront an insurmountable problem—many of the products lack ingredient labels and those that list ingredients do not adequately explain what they are. How is the average parent or art teacher to determine whether benzidine or cellulose ethyl hydroxyethyl ester poses a potential hazard to their child? In fact, the former is a potent human carcinogen, while the other is a harmless chemical used as a laxative.
>
> Exposure to art materials containing hazardous substances is not a small problem. According to the New York State Education Department's Bureau of Visual Arts and Humanities, approximately one million children were enrolled in art classes in the state's schools during the 1980–81 academic year.

In the investigation of art supplies in 15 New York school systems, representing 39% of the total enrollment of public school students in New York State, these kinds of chemical poisons were found:

Lead and Lead Compounds
These were found in "a wide range" of materials "including ceramic glazes, stained glass materials and pigments." Children "may develop lead poisoning after exposure to a small quantity of lead," the report noted, also citing a *New England Journal of Medicine* article showing children of lead workers "had contracted lead poisoning merely from coming in contact with their parents' workclothes. Lead is a carcinogen and

teratogen. There are several forms of exposure. Yet in the schools the tubes of Grumbacher Flake White Oil Paint—which contain 79% lead carbonate—only said "CONTAINS LEAD: HARMFUL IF EATEN."

Cadmium and Chromium
Both are suspected carcinogens. Cadmium and cadmium compounds were found in silver solders, paint pigments, ceramic glazes and fluxes. Chromium was found in pigments including chromium oxide green, strontium yellow, veridian, zinc yellow and chrome yellow.

Manganese Dioxide
The chemical, which can cause chronic manganese poisoning the symptoms of which are similar to Parkinson's Disease, was present in paint pigments including manganese blue, manganese violet, burnt umber, raw umber, Mars black and Mars brown.

Cobalt
Cobalt compounds are suspected carcinogens and were found in cerulean blue, cobalt blue and ultramarine blue pigments in the New Temp acrylics, Hyplar acrylics, Grumbacher oil paints and Liquetex acrylics found in most of the school systems.

Formaldehyde
Formaldehyde, a carcinogen, is used as a preservative in Academy water colors, New Temp acrylics, Liquetex acrylics and Hyplar acrylics.

In clays and glazes found in the schools, "an abundance of chronically toxic chemicals" was found—from silica which may produce silicosis, a respiratory disease, to fluorspar which can harm the lungs. Substances not listed on labels but also thought to be in the clays and glazes ranged from beryllium and nickel compounds, suspected carcinogens, to uranium which "may expose children to harmful radiation."

Among solvents which are toxic, the probe found six of the school systems using Krylon Crystal Clear Spray Coating which contains toluene which is linked to central nervous system depression, dermatitis and irritation of the respiratory tract. Xylene "shares many of the same hazardous qualities as tuolene" and was found in "magic markers" used in the schools including Sanford's and Markette markers.

Methylene chloride, a teratogen, possible mutagen, and a cause of liver damage and pulmonary edema, was found in paint strippers, aerosol sprays and varnish removers in some schools.

The report also listed instant papier maché mixes containing lead and asbestos, a carcinogen, and inks containing carbon black pigment which has been connected to cancer of the lungs, sinuses and skin.

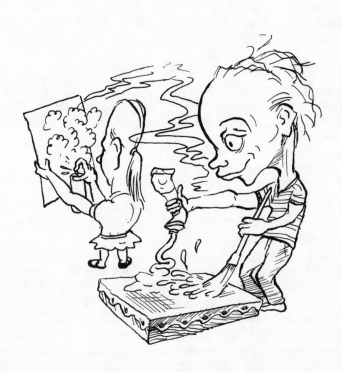

Because "cancer is a latent disease . . . it is highly unlikely that it would reveal clinically observable manifestations" in children. "Still, the risk to children using toxic art supplies is worth worrying about," the report asserted, because "no exposure" to a cancer-causing substance "is risk-free and the impact of repeated exposures may be culmulative. In addition, children are more susceptible to adverse health effects than adults—because they weigh less and have faster metabolisms, greater amounts of toxics may accumulate in their bodies than in adults' after comparable exposures. Also, the immunity and defense systems of children are not fully developed and are more vulnerable to toxic chemicals."

The Assembly committee declared:

> This investigation of toxic art and craft materials used in school systems in New York State found significant cause for concern regarding their impact on children's health. Art supplies containing powerful carcinogens and other potent, chronically toxic chemicals are commonly ordered for use in New York State classrooms.
>
> Art supplies, because they are used for pleasure and recreation, and because almost everyone has used them during childhood, are not thought of as potentially hazardous materials. However, as has been noted in this report, *many of them must be handled with extreme caution, because they contain chronically toxic chemicals*. Schools, in order to protect the health of their students, need information about the formulae of art and craft products they purchase. This can only be realized if product labels list chronically toxic ingredients and health precautions.

It demanded a "statuatory labeling standard for arts and crafts materials containing chronically toxic materials," labeling which would provide: 1) a statement of potential carcinogenicity or ability to cause long-term illness; 2) a listing of possibly chronically toxic ingredients; 3) a statement of the potential chronic health risks; 4) safe use and storage instructions; 5) a statement on where to obtain more health information (i.e., local poison control center); and, 6) the manufacturer's name and address.

But a bill providing for such standards failed in the New York State Legislature after issuance of the report. Earlier, a similar bill was defeated in the California Legislature, says McCann.

"There was a lot of lobbying by industry, particularly big industry, the paint industry, which was afraid," he says, "of having a precedent established increasing its liability."

The Many Love Canals

"We are facing a national chemical nightmare and this administration is treating it like a joke," Congressman James J. Florio of New Jersey, who heads a House subcommittee which is supposed to oversee the Environmental Protection Agency, declared in 1981.

Indeed, under Ronald Reagan the situation went from bad to worse. But for decades, under a pretense of protection, poisons have been dumped willy-nilly across America—and in recent years the early results have become manifest in illness and death.

Florio made his charges with release of a report showing, as Florio accurately phrased it, the EPA "is failing to protect the public health and environment from hazardous industrial wastes."

"Hundreds of potential Love Canals continue to operate," he said. "Millions of tons of hazardous wastes, including some that cause cancer, continue to be disposed of improperly. Public drinking water is threatened because industrial wastes are seeping into groundwater."

Five years before, Congress had passed the Resource Conservation and Recovery Act, a law directing EPA to take action against the dumping of hazardous wastes. "Yet EPA's response is to fill up a few dusty file drawers with some meaningless bureaucratic forms and pretend the whole problem will go away," said Florio. The General Accounting Office report "confirms what many of us have already suspected, namely that the current hazardous waste management system is stagnant, and provides little assurance that public health and the environment are protected." And, in fact, "federal assurance of public health protection and control over this nation's hazardous waste management system is virtually non-existent."

Here's the GAO report made at the request of Florio, chairman of the House Subcommittee on Commerce, Transportation and Tourism:

REPORT BY THE
Comptroller General
OF THE UNITED STATES

Hazardous Waste Facilities With Interim Status May Be Endangering Public Health And The Environment

The Environmental Protection Agency (EPA) has little assurance that hazardous waste facilities with interim status -- the period between application and issuance of the final permit -- meet the minimum national requirements for acceptable management as specified in the interim status regulations. In addition, all facilities are not included in the interim status process.

Interim status regulations are largely administrative and do not specify the kinds of technical, design, construction, and operating requirements needed for health and environmental protection.

EPA and State inspection and enforcement efforts have covered only a small percentage of the facilities with interim status. EPA has emphasized the issuance of warning letters, notices of violations, and compliance orders which, due to the nature of the regulations, have concentrated on administrative violations.

Most EPA and State officials believe that additional staffing is necessary to implement a more comprehensive interim status program for hazardous waste facilities.

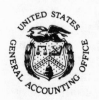

CED-81-158
SEPTEMBER 28, 1981

Of an estimated 30,000 hazardous waste treatment, storage and disposal facilities in the U.S., operators of only 14,700 submitted the EPA's required "interim status" application and the "EPA made little effort" to find out about the others, the report found.

Said the report:

ALL HAZARDOUS WASTE FACILITIES ARE NOT REGULATED AND

REGULATED FACILITIES MAY NOT MEET REQUIREMENTS

RCRA provides that facilities which store, treat, or dispose of hazardous waste may obtain interim status, and EPA requires that facilities with interim status must meet the interim status regulations and requirements. However, compliance with interim status regulations is not a condition for a facility to obtain interim status.

EPA has little assurance that all facilities which store, treat or dispose of hazardous waste were "captured" by the interim status process or that those facilities with interim status meet the interim status regulations and requirements because:

  --Generators which handle small amounts of hazardous waste were not required by EPA to obtain interim status.

  --EPA has performed little followup to determine if all existing hazardous waste facilities, required by regulations submitted applications.

  --The interim status application process was not designed to determine compliance with the regulations and requirements.

Information noted in the interim status applications reviewed raises questions about interim status facility compliance with the regulations and requirements. Also, our visits to 38 interim status facilities and review of EPA inspection reports showed that most interim status facilities did not meet the regulations and requirements.

In a sampling of facilities which did have EPA approval for "interim status," 29 out of 38 showed "instances of noncompliance."

Some examples given by the GAO:

Chromium lead sludge disposal

One facility we visited was annually depositing an estimated
4,560 tons of chromium lead sludge directly into a 40-acre body
of water. Although this area bordered on a lake connected to
Lake Michigan and had been classified by a Federal agency as
a "wetland" area requiring special preservation, the facility
had not obtained the required Clean Water Act operating permit.
In addition, although the facility was classified as a hazardous waste landfill it had not obtained the necessary State permit and therefore was in violation of State hazardous waste management regulations. The State inspector who accompanied us
agreed with our observations. The facility had interim status
under RCRA.

Phenol disposal

At another facility, wastewater with a concentration of
117 to 135 parts per million (ppm) of a hazardous substance
called phenol was being discharged directly onto the land. EPA
water quality criteria prescribe a maximum tolerable level for
human consumption of 3.5 ppm. The State inspector acknowledged
that the practice looked improper, yet the company's Part A application for interim status and the information filed at the
EPA regional office provided no indication that this type of
hazardous waste activity was taking place. This facility also
had interim status under RCRA.

Polychlorinated biphenyl (PCB)
burning and disposal problems

At another location visited the facility was involved
in incinerating PCB's, a highly toxic hazardous waste subject to
various special regulations. Personnel operating the facility,
as well as the inspector accompanying us, could provide no assur-
ances of the adequacy of the burning temperatures--according
to EPA, from 1,200 degrees to 1,600 degrees centigrade were required. The cinder residues remaining were also being disposed
of directly on the ground beside the incinerator with no special
physical controls. This facility also had interim status.

Chemical surface impoundment
problems

A chemical surface impoundment facility did not have a
protective cover or enough freeboard around the facility to prevent wind and water erosion. We observed run-off from the facility which extended past the firm's property lines. Although the
EPA inspector agreed with our observations regarding the facility,
the facility had interim status under RCRA.

The report flatly concluded that the EPA was not providing
"for protection of public health and the environment."

The GAO report is one of a number of government reports
on how we have been dumping huge amounts of poisons onto
the earth behind a façade of protection.

In 1979, the House Subcommittee on Oversight and Investigations issued this report:

HAZARDOUS WASTE DISPOSAL

REPORT

together with

ADDITIONAL AND SEPARATE VIEWS

BY THE

SUBCOMMITTEE ON OVERSIGHT AND INVESTIGATIONS

OF THE

COMMITTEE ON INTERSTATE AND FOREIGN COMMERCE

HOUSE OF REPRESENTATIVES

NINETY-SIXTH CONGRESS

FIRST SESSION

SEPTEMBER 1979

Said the panel's chairman on the report's opening page:

Inadequate disposal of hundreds of billions of pounds of hazardous
waste at both active and inactive sites poses severe threats to man and
the environment. Millions of people are exposed to toxic materials leaking from these sites. Evidence presented to the Subcommittee indicates
that people living near disposal sites may face not only immediate adverse health effects, but the potential for higher risk of disease in the
future.

The Subcommittee is very concerned over the failure of the Environmental Protection Agency (EPA), industry and the Congress
to meet the challenge presented by hazardous waste disposal. EPA has
failed to meet statutory deadlines for regulations on disposal of hazardous wastes; has failed to determine the location of all hazardous
waste sites; and has not taken vigorous enforcement actions. Industry
has, in many cases, continued inadequate disposal practices long after
they had knowledge that these practices were resulting in water and
land contamination. And the Congress has allocated far too few funds
to deal effectively with a problem of this magnitude.

> BOB ECKHARDT,
> *Chairman, Subcommittee on*
> *Oversight and Investigations.*

Then came a segment of the testimony of an assistant U.S.
attorney general:

HAZARDOUS WASTE DISPOSAL

"I believe that it is probably the first or second most serious environmental problem in the country. One of the difficulties is that we really
do not know what the dimensions of the problem are. Essentially,
there is very little downside risk to anybody who illegally disposes of
chemicals in such a way as to be harmful to the public health.

We do not know where the millions of tons of stuff is going. We feel
that the things that have turned up like the Love Canal and Kin-Buc
situation are simply the tip of the iceberg. We do not have the capacity
at this time really to find out what is actually happening. In my view,
it is simply a wide open situation, like the Wild West was in the 1870's,
for toxic disposal.

The public is basically unprotected. There just are not any lawmen
out there, State or Federal, policing this subject."

> JAMES MOORMAN, *Assistant Attorney General for Land and*
> *Natural Resources, U.S. Department of Justice,* in testi-
> mony before the Subcommittee on Oversight and Investi-
> gations, May 16, 1979.

The public is basically unprotected. There just are not any lawmen out there, State or Federal, policing this subject.

Stressed the Subcommittee's report:

The hazardous waste disposal problem cannot be overstated. The Environmental Protection Agency (EPA) has estimated that 77,140,-000,000 pounds of hazardous waste are generated each year, but only 10 percent of that amount is disposed of in an environmentally sound manner.[1] Today, there are some 30,000 hazardous waste disposal sites in the United States.[2] Because of years of inadequate disposal practices and the absence of regulation, hundreds and perhaps thousands of these sites now pose an imminent hazard to man and the environment. Our country presently lacks an adequate program to determine where these sites are; to clean up unsafe active and inactive sites; and to provide sufficient facilities for the safe disposal of hazardous wastes in the future.

We have investigated environmental contamination resulting from disposal sites in all areas of the country; from the Love Canal in New York to the Valley of the Drums in Shepardsville, Kentucky, to Lathrop, California. We have found that massive quantities of chemical and pesticide waste contaminants as well as other toxic materials are leaking out of disposal sites or "non-sites" where waste has been illegally dumped in open fields, swamps, and vacant lots. It also has been spread on roads as a dangerous ingredient of road oil. In sum, the Subcommittee finds that proper disposal of hazardous materials is the exception, rather than the rule.

Federal and State efforts to control disposal of hazardous wastes are totally inadequate. With adoption of the Resource Conservation and Recovery Act (RCRA) in the fall of 1976, Congress established for the first time a Federal program to regulate the disposal of hazardous wastes. While the Congress may have been unrealistic in giving EPA only 18 months to develop national standards for the proper disposal of these wastes, there can be no excuse for EPA's failure to promulgate regulations in the nearly three years since the statute was enacted. EPA also has failed to conduct a comprehensive search for hazardous waste sites and to pursue enforcement actions vigorously.

It must also be said that industry has shown laxity, not infrequently to the point of criminal negligence, in soiling the land and adulterating the waters with its toxins. And it cannot be denied that Congress has shown lethargy in legislating controls and appropriating funds for their enforcement.

As a result, even an extraordinary effort, commenced immediately, cannot achieve adequate protection for the American public for years to come. In the interim, it is our duty—that is, the government's duty—to sound a warning. That is what your Subcommittee is doing here.

It issued these findings:

II. SUMMARY OF FINDINGS AND RECOMMENDATIONS

A. FINDINGS

1. FINDINGS CONCERNING DISPOSAL OF HAZARDOUS WASTE

(a) *Common characteristics of dump sites*

The Subcommittee investigation of over one dozen hazardous waste disposal problems revealed four characteristics that were common to most of the sites:

(1) The sites contain large quantities of hazardous waste:

—Hooker Chemical's three disposal sites in the Niagara Falls, New York, area contain an estimated 352 million pounds of industrial chemical waste, including TCP (which is often contaminated with one of the most toxic substances known to man, dioxin) and lindane, a highly toxic pesticide product.

—Occidental Chemical Company's site at Lathrop, California, discharged thousands of gallons of pesticide formulation wastes into the ground on the company site.

—Hooker dumped millions of pounds of hazardous wastes in the local municipal dumps on Long Island, New York.

—The Valley of the Drums in Shepardsville, Kentucky, contains over 17,000 barrels of hazardous wastes.

—The Chemical Control site in Elizabeth, New Jersey, contained over 40,000 barrels of hazardous wastes. At least 100 pounds of picric acid, a powerful explosive, also was found stored on the site.

(2) Unsafe design and disposal methods are widespread:

—At the S-Area site in Niagara Falls, drums of liquid hazardous wastes were rolled into trenches and tank wagons were discharged directly into pits at a site composed of reclaimed land. Samples of sediment from a water treatment plant only a few hundred feet from the site suggest that chemicals from the dump site have entered the water supply.

—A similar disposal method at the Hardeman County, Tennessee site resulted in the contamination of well water.

—At the Valley of the Drums, thousands of barrels were stacked illegally in the hauler's backyard. These drums are in a seriously deteriorating state, and some have already burst and spilled their contents on the ground.

—At Hooker's Montague, Michigan site, barrels of hazardous waste were often dumped off the backs of trucks and hacked open by men armed with axes. The nature of the area affords no geological protection against the wastes reaching local groundwater.

—At the Elizabeth, New Jersey site, tens of thousands of barrels of highly toxic, explosive and flammable materials are unsafely "stored" within a few feet of the Company's waste incinerator, within a few feet of a local road and a railroad right of way and within one quarter mile of huge liquified natural gas and propane storage tanks.

—At Lathrop, California, pesticide formulation waste products placed in lagoons were allowed to percolate into the extremely permeable soil, threatening the area's drinking and irrigation water.

—In Denver, Colorado, radioactive waste products from old radium industry operations have been discovered throughout the Denver area.

—In Central Florida, hundreds of homes were built on land covered with waste containing radium and thorium from old phosphate operations; unhealthy levels of radon gas have been found in hundreds of homes.

—At the Love Canal, the safety of clay-lined landfills for disposal of highly toxic organic waste has been questioned.

—Waste oil contaminated with toxic chemicals was laid on 9 roads in East Texas due to the negligence of the waste disposal company.

(3) The danger to the environment is substantial:

—Contaminated groundwater has rendered unusable the local water supplies in Montague, Michigan; Lathrop, California; parts of two counties on Long Island, including the towns of Bethpage and Glenn Cove; and around the dump site in Hardeman County, Tennessee.

—Leachate from the S-area dump threatens the principal water supply of the City of Niagara Falls.

—Two hundred thirty families have been evacuated from the Love Canal and the property values of the entire neighborhood have been rendered negligible.

(4) Many sites pose major health hazards:

—The Love Canal health data shows elevated miscarrage and birth defect rates; evidence suggests many other health effects, the nature and extent of which are in dispute.

—Excessive radiation levels in Denver, Colorado, and Central Florida pose serious risks of latent cancers and genetic damage. For example, EPA has estimated that the Florida area residents' risk of contracting lung cancer is 35 percent above average.

—The State of New Jersey has estimated that a fire or explosion at the Chemical Control site could produce a toxic cloud of chemicals that could threaten hundreds of thousands of people in the New York metropolitan area.

(b) Inadequate State and local response to threats to the public health from hazardous waste disposal:

—The Board of Education of Niagara Falls permitted a public school to be built on top of the Love Canal site and local officials permitted a residential subdivision to be built adjacent to the site.

—The New York State Health Department has failed to assure residents of the Love Canal that the public health is being adequately protected.

—The Orange District Office of the Texas Department of Water Resources did not perform an adequate investigation of contaminated road oil dumped in East Texas and, therefore, failed to discover a potential public health problem until after any damage was already done.

(c) The failure to properly dispose of hazardous waste is costing the public millions and the cost of cleanup is far more expensive than proper disposal in the first place:

—An EPA report estimates that it will cost between $13.1 and $22.1 billion to clean up all hazardous waste that pose a danger to public health and the environment.

—Cleanup costs at the Love Canal have already exceeded $27 million and area residents are seeking more than $2 billion for personal injury and property damage. It is estimated that a properly secured disposal site would have cost only $4 million (in 1979 dollars) in 1952 when the site was closed.

—The State of Michigan has estimated the cost of cleaning up the Montague site at $100 million.

—The State of New Jersey has estimated the cost of cleaning up Chemical Control at $10 million.

—EPA estimates it will cost up to $2.9 million for remedial work to eliminate the danger of phosphate slag in Florida.

—The Colorado Health Department says that cleaning up the radium in Denver could cost up to $25 million.

—Should the containment efforts at the S-area in Niagara Falls and on Long Island fail, the cost of building alternative water supply systems would be astronomical.

(d) Special problems with certain kinds of dump sites:

—Abandoned sites—those where no owner can be found or where the owner cannot afford the cost of clean up—have forced State and local governments to bear the costs.

—On-site facilities—those owned and operated by the generators of the waste, either on the plant site or elsewhere—pose serious problems because State regulation of them historically has been minimal. The Subcommittee's survey of the 53 largest domestic chemical manufacturers revealed that 94% of their wastes have been disposed of on the plant site.

(e) Locating future sites will be difficult:

—The Nation is facing a critical storage of safe disposal sites for hazardous wastes which will be exacerbated as hazardous waste production increases.

(1) The State of New Jersey testified that it is having difficulty finding a home for the more than 40,000 barrels of chemicals at the Chemical Control site.

(2) The State of Kentucky has not yet located a safe home

for the 17,000 partially buried drums at the Valley of the
Drums.

(3) The Colorado Department of Health is having difficulty finding a disposal site for the 70,000 cubic feet of
radium-contaminated soil in Denver.

"The Love Canal is the most well-known of the problem
sites," said the report, but . . .

The Hyde Park site also raised serious public health concerns. The
toxins emanating from the dump via Bloody Run Creek have caused
serious respiratory problems for a large family, the Armagosts, according to testimony from their physician. Local union representatives
from the plants adjoining the dump gave extensive testimony on
the health problems experienced by the workers, particularly respiratory and skin problems, including cancer. Many of the acute symptoms
coincided with exposure to toxic fumes given off by the dump site.
Responding to requests by Chairman Eckhardt as well as the United
Steelworkers of America and the Oil, Chemical and Atomic Workers
International Union, the National Institute of Occupational Safety
and Health (NIOSH) promptly initiated a comprehensive health
hazard evaluation of the workers in those three plants. The results
of that survey are not yet available.

Among the 16.5 million gallons of compounds dumped by Velsicol
at the Hardeman County, Tennessee site were endrin, heptachlor,
benzene, and aldrin, all carcinogens or suspected carcinogens.

The following quotation from the 1972 State order closing the dump
site clearly indicates that this land may never again be usable:

The dangers presented by these compounds are directly related
to their high toxicity and persistent toxicity over long periods of
time.

The characteristics of these compounds which create a danger
to both man and the environment include extreme toxicity over
long periods of time, indicating very slow degradation; near insolubility in water with the tendency to cling or adhere to particulate matter; and the ability to accumulate in the fatty tissues of
most animals and to be absorbed by vegetable crops from contaminated soil, thereby entering man's feed chain.

Due to the compounds' insolubility and cling characteristics, the
water becomes a mover of the wastes.

Local residents' drinking water near the Hardeman County dump
site was found to contain at least a dozen dangerous pesticide manufacturing wastes. The levels of carbon tetrachloride in a nearby drinking
water well, for example, was 48 times that found in the Ohio River
when Cincinnati residents were warned not to drink the water.

Drinking water contamination in Montague, Michigan, Long Island, New York, and Lathrop, California, pose potential long-run health problems for affected residents. Chronic exposure to low levels of toxic chemicals may produce health problems which may not be known for years due to long latency periods.

The Chemical Control site poses a toxic, explosive, and fire hazard to the residents of both Northern New Jersey and New York City, despite the fact that the State of New Jersey has removed the picric acid. The State has estimated that fire or explosion on this site could spread and possibly ignite millions of gallons of liquid natural gas stored within a quarter of a mile of the site. The resulting fire and explosion could injure thousands of people.

Additionally, a fire or explosion at the site itself could produce a toxic cloud of chemicals which could drift for miles threatening hundreds of thousands of people.

And where has the protection been?

B. Inadequate State and Local Response to Threats to the Public Health From Hazardous Waste Disposal

Just as EPA has not effectively exercised its imminent hazard authority under RCRA, State and local agencies have either failed to recognize or been unable to take appropriate action to protect adequately against threats to the public health from hazardous waste disposal.

In certain cases, officials were either woefully uninformed or derelict in their duty. For example, the Board of Education of the City of Niagara Falls chose to build a public school on top of the Love Canal dump site, and then local officials permitted a residential subdivision to be built immediately adjacent to the site. While it is difficult to believe that the School Board fully understood the composition and potential danger of the waste materials, the deed conveying the property from Hooker to the School Board did include a warning that chemicals were stored in the Canal. In undocumented testimony, Hooker claimed that the School Board was warned against construction activity of any kind and deeded the property only upon the insistence of the Board. Clearly, the victims of the Love Canal disaster have reason to question whether State and local officials have committed themselves to a maximum effort to minimize the danger to the public health.

Look at this interchange involving Senator Albert Gore and a Hooker Chemical official:

Hooker Chemical was aware at least as early as 1958 that children were experiencing chemical burns from substances percolating up from the Love Canal dump site yet took no action to inform local residents of the potential hazards. Mr. Wilkenfeld, formerly of Hooker Chemical, was questioned on this point:

Mr. GORE. Twenty-one years ago when this incident occurred with the children being burned, did the company warn only the school board or did you take any steps to alert the people who lived there?

Mr. WILKENFELD. It was my understanding that the people who lived in the area knew that this was a former chemical dump and that these materials were hazardous and that the children should not get in there.

As a matter of fact, on these occasions when children would get into material like that, they quite frequently would call our plant dispensary to get information from the nurse on treatment of irritation from the chemicals.

Mr. GORE. Did you tell them not to play in the area?

Mr. WILKENFELD. I can't say what the nurse's response was.

Mr. GORE. Did you take any steps to inform the people who lived adjacent to the Love Canal dump site to inform them of what kinds of chemicals were in the dump site and what the hazards to their health were?

Mr. WILKENFELD. No; we did not.

Mr. GORE. Why not?

Meanwhile, Hooker was trying to sell off another contaminated dump site—and throughout it all, Hooker's relationship with local officials was most cozy:

Nor was Hooker sufficiently concerned with the potential health problems posed by the Love Canal to keep the Company from contemplating the disposal of another site—the 102nd Street dump—in a similar manner. A 1972 internal Hooker memo suggests three possible uses for that site: sale to the city of Niagara Falls; sale or lease to private interests for development (the land had been zoned as multiple family residential); or use by Hooker as a warehouse. Another memo suggested that the City of Niagara Falls might want to buy the land for park and recreational facilities.

It is obvious from the testimony surrounding each of the Niagara Falls sites that the relationship between Hooker and local officials was very cooperative. Mr. Robert Matthews, Director of Utilities for the City of Niagara Falls and the individual charged with responsibility for the water intake system that is threatened by the migration of toxic chemicals from the S-Area site, volunteered his opinion of the relationship between Hooker and the City:

Insofar as my experience is concerned—and, again, it is limited to water and waste water in Niagara Falls—Hooker has acted very responsibly. Hooker executives have given me good and learned advice. When you are in a situation such as I am in, you need advice.

There are further GAO reports on the subject, like this one:

REPORT BY THE
Comptroller General
OF THE UNITED STATES

Hazardous Waste Sites Pose Investigation, Evaluation, Scientific, And Legal Problems

Not much is known about the possible adverse health and environmental effects associated with the thousands of hazardous waste disposal sites now being discovered throughout the United States.

The Environmental Protection Agency is finding it difficult to carry out its mandate to protect human health and the environment from hazardous wastes because:

  --New waste sites are being discovered faster than they can be investigated and evaluated.

  --There is no strong scientific basis for determining risks.

  --Legal action seeking correction of hazardous waste problems is pursued for only a few sites.

Individuals seeking relief within the courts to satisfy hazardous waste compensation claims face great difficulties.

New "superfund" legislation will provide some help, but it is too early to tell whether it will solve all of the problems presented by uncontrolled hazardous waste sites.

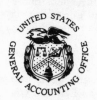

CED-81-57
APRIL 24, 1981

It concluded:

D I G E S T

Existing legislation authorizes a program of
grants to States and territories to develop
solid waste management plans for the recovery
of energy and other resources from discarded
materials, the safe disposal of discarded
materials, and the management of hazardous
wastes. The law also required the Environmental Protection Agency (EPA) to establish
criteria for classifying all land disposal
facilities as either environmentally acceptable or unacceptable and for participating
States to evaluate facilities against the
criteria and to report the results to EPA.
EPA was to publish an inventory of all
unacceptable facilities or "open dumps"
identified according to the criteria.

At the request of Congressman Albert Gore, Jr.,
GAO reviewed the status of State solid waste
management plans, the conduct of the open-dump
inventory, and the impact of reduced funding
on State solid waste activities.

Over $47 million was awarded to States from
October 1977 to March 1981 to develop State
solid waste management plans and to conduct an
open-dump inventory. Plan development, however, has been slow. No State plans have
been approved by EPA as of June 1981. The
open-dump inventory published by EPA in late
May 1981 is incomplete and is not the management tool intended to apprise the Congress
and the public of the overall magnitude of
solid waste land disposal problems throughout
the Nation.

And note this subsequent GAO report:

BY THE U.S. GENERAL ACCOUNTING OFFICE
Report To The Honorable Albert Gore, Jr. House Of Representatives

Solid Waste Disposal Practices:
--Open Dumps Not Identified
--States Face Funding Problems

In 1976 the Resource Conservation and Recovery Act was passed to deal with, among other things, the Nation's open-dumping problem and the lack of a national solid waste management program. Some problems this law was intended to correct still exist because:

> --The Environmental Protection Agency has been slow to develop guidelines and approve State solid waste management plans.

> --EPA's May 1981 open-dump inventory does not provide an overview of the magnitude of the Nation's solid waste disposal problems.

EPA's proposed fiscal year 1982 budget includes no funding for the States' solid waste activities. Since they lack other sources of funds, States predict solid waste problems will persist.

GAO is recommending actions to develop a complete open-dump inventory and to encourage alternative funding sources for State solid waste management programs.

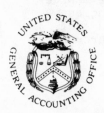

CED-81-131
JULY 23, 1981

It concluded:

D̲ I̲ G̲ E̲ S̲ T̲

Hazardous waste sites have been referred to as
"ticking time bombs" with the potential to cause
untold damage to human health and the environment. The Environmental Protection Agency (EPA)
is charged by the Resource Conservation and Recovery Act with protecting human health and the
environment from these wastes.

To carry out this mandate, EPA is to (1) discover, investigate, evaluate, and respond to
uncontrolled hazardous waste sites, 1/ (2) perform hazardous waste research, and (3) seek
solutions to hazardous waste problems and, if
necessary, file suit in Federal courts.

EPA has had difficulty in fully performing these
activities for a number of reasons. For example,
EPA's

--site investigation and evaluation activities lag behind an ever-increasing number
  of potential sites requiring investigation
  and evaluation (see ch. 2),

--capabilities to identify and analyze hazardous waste and understand the real or potential risk these wastes pose to human
  health and the environment are limited by
  both cost and scientific knowledge (see
  ch. 3), and

--past enforcement and cleanup efforts were
  limited by resources required to demonstrate potential harm in a court case and
  by the need to identify financially
  viable defendants (individuals or companies) to pay for remedial measures
  or cleanup costs. (See pp. 36 to 39.)

*. . . 'ticking time bombs' with the potential to cause untold
damage to human health and the environment . . . yet The
Environmental Protection Agency is finding it difficult to
carry out its mandate. . .*

As to *what should be done*, all the investigations emphasize
a need for stricter laws and penalties including strengthened
criminal penalties but say that equally important must be the
will on the part of would-be protectors to do their jobs.

"The Federal and State governments are not powerless to
combat the problem of hazardous waste disposal," said the
House Subcommittee on Oversight and Investigations. It is
just somehow that they won't and don't.

Spreading It Around

With America producing so many toxic substances and encumbered with so much toxic waste, U.S. corporations have been working to ship toxic wastes to nations in the Caribbean, South America, Africa and Asia—to dump the tons upon tons of poisons there. Meanwhile, the U.S. is at the base of a gigantic international network of poison trade.

It took eight months to obtain, through the U.S. Freedom of Information Act, information about the global toxic waste-dumping scheme from the U.S. government. Here are some of the documents involving the plan.

This 1981 State Department dispatch was sent to these U.S. embassies—all in countries which the project could involve:

```
HARRIS LAWRENCE T          12/14/81 190443   PRINTER: LI
80 STATE 37348
                      UNCLASSIFIED
UNCLASSIFIED
PAGE 01         STATE   037348
ORIGIN OES-09
INFO  OCT-00  ADS-00  SIG-03  COMF-00  CEQ-01  EPAE-00
      ACDA-12  CIAE-00  INR-10  IO-15  L-03  NSAE-00  NSC-05
      EB-08  ARC-22  DODE-00  E-02  DOE-17  SS-15  SP-02
      PM-05  SAS-02  HEW-06  DLOS-09  AID-07  NSF-02  ICA-15
      INT-05  FMC-02  CG-00  DOTE-00  AF-10  ARA-15  EA-12
      EUR-12  NEA-07  AIT-02  AGR-01  SPH-01  '217 R
DRAFTED BY CES/ENH:JSARTORIUS
APPROVED BY OES/ENH:DRKING
OES/E:WHAYNE
EUR/RPE:LMORSE
COMMERCE/OEA - OPAYNTER
```

```
AF/EPS - CABRYANT
CEQ - BHBAAS
NEA/ECON - RFGRAHAM
EPA/OIA - DOAKLEY
ARA/ECP - CALLEN
                     ------------------032935  130132Z /15 46
R 122030Z FEB 80
FM SECSTATE WASHDC
TO AIOECD
AMEMBASSY COTONOU
AMEMBASSY RABAT
AMEMBASSY YAOUNDE
AMEMBASSY.BRAZZAVILLE
MEMBASSY LIBREVILLE 2320-232--2322-2323
AMEMBASSY BANJUL
AMEMBASSY ACCRA
AMEMBASSY CONAKRY
AMEMBASSY BISSAU
AMEMBASSY ABIDJAN
AMEMBASSY MONROVIA
AMEMBASSY LAGOS
AMEMBASSY KINSHASA
UNCLASSIFIED
UNCLASSIFIED
PAGE 02          STATE   037348
AMEMBASSY NOUAKCHOTT
AMEMBASSY DAKAR
AMEMBASSY LOME
AMEMBASSY PRAIA
AMEMBASSY BUENOS AIRES
AMEMBASSY BRASILIA
AMEMBASSY BOGOTA
AMEMBASSY QUITO
AMEMBASSY GEORGETOWN
AMEMBASSY LIMA
AMEMBASSY PARAMARIBO
AMEMBASSY MONTEVIDEO
AMEMBASSY CARACAS
AMEMBASSY MEXICO
AMEMBASSY SAN JOSE
AMCONSUL BELIZE
AMEMBASSY SAN SALVADOR
AMEMBASSY GUATEMALA
AMEMBASSY MANAGUA
AMEMBASSY TEGUCIGALPA
AMEMBASSY PANAMA
AMEMBASSY NASSAU
AMEMBASSY BRIDGETOWN
AMEMBASSY SANTO DOMINGO
AMEMBASSY PORT AU PRINCE
AMCONSUL CURACAO
AMEMBASSY KINGSTON
AMCONSUL MARTINIQUE
AMEMBASSY PORT OF SPAIN
AMEMBASSY TOKYO
AMEMBASSY RANGOON
AMEMBASSY JAKARTA
AMEMBASSY SEOUL
```

```
AMEMBASSY KUALA LUMPUR
AMEMBASSY MANILA
AMEMBASSY PORT MORESBY
AMEMBASSY BANGKOK
AMEMBASSY ALGIERS
AMEMBASSY CAIRO
AMEMBASSY TUNIS
AMEMBASSY ANKARA
AMEMBASSY DAMASCUS
USMISSION USUN NEW YORK
USMISSION GENEVA
INFO AMEMBASSY FREETOWN
AMEMBASSY NAIROBI
AMEMBASSY SANTIAGO
```

As the State Department described the situation:

```
SUBJECT:      EXPORTS OF HAZARDOUS (NON-NUCLEAR) WASTES
BEGIN SUMMARY:  FACED WITH INCREASING COSTS AND GOVERNMENT
REGULATORY CONTROLS ASSOCIATED WITH THE DISPOSAL OF
HAZARDOUS (NON-NUCLEAR) WASTES IN THE U.S., SOME
AMERICAN COMPANIES ARE NOW CONSIDERING DISPOSAL SITES IN
DEVELOPING COUNTRIES.  THIS COULD RESULT IN N A ORABLE
ENVIRONMENTAL/HEALTH EFFECTS IN LDCS, AND ADVERSE FOREIGN
AND DOMESTIC PUBLIC CONCERN.  POSTS ARE REQUESTED TO
REPORT ON DEVELOPMENTS THAT BEAR ON THIS ISSUE, WHICH ARE
EITHER CURRENTLY TAKING PLACE OR MAY COME TO YOUR ATTENTION
IN THE FUTURE.  THE NEED FOR SUCH REPORTS FROM WEST AFRICAN
AND CARIBBEAN POSTS IS PARTICULARLY URGENT.  END SUMMARY.


PAGE 04         STATE  237348
1. AT PRESENT THERE IS INSUFFICIENT TECHNICAL KNOWLEDGE
OF HOW TO STORE, DISPOSE OF, OR REPROCESS SAFELY MANY
HAZARDOUS WASTES GENERATED BY AMERICAN INDUSTRY.  ONE
SOLUTION, THE DESTRUCTION OR NEUTRALIZATION OF SUCH
WASTES, MANY OF WHICH ARE LONG-LIVED AND TOXIC, IS PROV-
ING TO BE EXPENSIVE AND DIFFICULT.  ANOTHER SOLUTION,
LOG-TERM CONTAINMENT STORAGE (FOR EXAMPLE, IN MINES OR
EVEN IN DRUMS OR BURIED IN THE GROUND) IS ALSO EXPENSIVE
(BECAUSE OF ONGOING MONITORING AND MANAGEMENT COSTS) AND
OFTEN PRESENTS SERIOUS HEALTH AND ENVIRONMENTAL HAZARDS
BECAUSE THE CONTAINERS OR WASTE SITES CAN EVENTUALLY FAIL,
WITH THE WASTES ENTERING GROUND WATER OR RUNNING OFF INTO
SURFACE WATER -- AFFECTING HUMAN HEALTH NOT ONLY THROUGH
WATER POTABILITY BUT ALSO BY EATING AGRICULTURAL PRODUCTS
AND FISH NURTURED BY, OR LIVING IN CONTAMINATED WATER.
FACED WITH THE PROBLEMS OF INCREASING COST OF DOMESTIC
RECOVERY AND AN INCREASING DISINCLINATION OF STATE AND
LOCAL JURISDICTIONS TO ALLOW EITHER TRANSPORTATION OR
RESOURCE RECOVERY DISPOSAL ACTIVITIES, AND THE NEW
RESOURCES CONSERVATION AND RECOVERY ACT PROCEDURES IMPLE-
MENTED BY THE ENVIRONMENTAL PROTECTION AGENCY (EPA), U.S.
```

```
INDUSTRY IS FINDING ITSELF HARD PRESSE  TO GET RID OF ITS
HAZARDOUS WASTES.  CONSEQUENTLY, A NUMBER OF AMERICAN
COMPANIES ARE NOW CONSIDERING SITES FOR ALL FORMS OF
HAZARDOUS (EXCEPT NUCLEAR) WASTES IN DEVELOPING COUN-
TRIES, WHERE SUCH PROPOSALS MAY BE WELCOMED AS PROVIDING
A SOURCE OF MUCH-NEEDED FOREIGN EXCHANGE.
```

The dispatch spoke of a move by the Nedlog Technology Group, Inc. of Arvada, Colorado to dump wastes in Sierra Leone in Africa—paying that nation $25 million a year.

The dispatch went on:

```
                              THE AFRICAN WEST COAST
HAS BECOME A PRIME TARGET FOR DISPOSING OF MILLIONS OF
TONS OF US WASTES, CITING PROPOSALS (IN ADDITION TO
SIERRA LEONE AND CHILE) IN NIGERIA, LIBERIA AND SENEGAL.
FURTHER, A PHILADELPHIA LANDFILL OWNER, DAVID EHRLICH,
CLAIMED HE HAD RECENTLY OBTAINED PERMISSION FROM ONE
COUNTRY ALONG THE AFRICAN WEST COAST, UNIDENTIFIED BUT
NOT SIERRA LEONE, TO SET UP A PROCESSING AND DISPOSAL
OPERATION FOR US CHEMICAL WASTES; HE PLANNED TO BE
DUMPING IN "SEVERAL WEEKS".  WE ALSO HAVE RUMORS THAT
A US COMPANY IS NEGOTIATING WITH THE GOVERNMENT OF HAITI
FOR WASTE DISPOSAL.
```

It declared:

```
7. CONSIDERING SHIPPING COSTS AND PROXIMITY TO MAJOR
HAZARDOUS WASTE PRODUCING COUNTRIES, THE FOLLOWING AREAS
APPEAR TO BE THE MOST LIKELY CANDIDATES FOR DISPOS L
SITES: WEST AFRICA. SOUTH AND CENTRAL AMERICA. THE
CARIBBEAN, EAST ASIA AND THE MEDITERRANEAN LITTORAL.
. ACTION: WEST AFRICAN AND CARIBBEAN POSTS, PARTICULARLY
LAGOS, MONROVIA, DAKAR AND PORT-AU-PRINCE ARE REQUESTED
TO REPORT SOONEST ANY INFORMATION THAT CAN BE DEVELOPED
CONFIRMING OR DENYING POSSIBLE APPROACHES OR CONTRACTS BY
US (AND OTHER) COMPANIES IN THE HAZARDOUS (NON-NUCLEAR
WASTE DISPOSAL FIELD.
```

This State Department dispatch to "all diplomatic and consular posts" was also sent in 1981:

```
R 141331Z JUL 81 ZEX
FM SECSTATE WASHDC
TO ALL DIPLOMATIC AND CONSULAR POSTS
UNCLAS STATE 184172
INFORM ALL CONSULS
E.O. 12065:  N/A
TAGS: SENV, ECON
SUBJECT: EXPORTS OF HAZARDOUS (NON-NUCLEAR) WASTE
REF: 80STATE 37348
1.  SUMMARY:  ON NOVEMBER 19, 1980, NEW REGULATIONS
UNCLASSIFIED
UNCLASSIFIED
PAGE 02        STATE  184172
GOVERNING TREATMENT, STORAGE, TRANSPORTATION, AND DISPOSAI
OF HAZARDOUS WASTES IN THE U.S. WENT INTO EFFE T.  THESE
REGULATIONS MAY INCREASE INTEREST IN EXPORTING WASTES
GENERATED IN THE U.S.  SOME AMERICAN COMPANIES MAY BE CON-
SIDERING DISPOSAL IN DEVELOPING, AS WELL AS DEVELOPED
```

```
5.  UNDER RCRA, THE U.S. HAS NO MEANS OF REGULATING THE
EXPORT OF HAZARDOUS WASTES.  HOWEVER, EPA AND THE DEPART-
MENT HAVEINSTITUTED A POLICY OF NOTIFYING THE POTENTIAL
RECIPIENT GOVERNMENT OF A PROPOSED EXPORT, BASED ON INFOR-
MATION PROVIDED BY THE U.S. WASTE GENERATOR IN THE REQUIR-
ED NOTIFICATION TO EPA.  THE NOTIFICATION MUST INCLUDE
THE NAME AND ADDRESS OF THE WASTE GENERATOR; THE NAME AND
ADDRESS OF THE FOREIGN CONSIGNEE; THE EPA WASTE IDEN IFI-
CATION NUMBER; AND THE DEPARTMENT OF TRANSPORTATION
SHIPPING DESCRIPTION (PROPER SHIPPING NAME, HAZARDOUS
CLASS AND UN NUMBER).  NOTIFICATION TO THE RECEIVING
COUNTRY IS DONE BY CABLE TO U.S. POSTS ABROAD REQUESTING
THAT THE INFORMATION CONTAINED THEREIN BE PASSED IMMEDI-
ATELY TO APPROPRIATE HOST COUNTRY OFFICIALS.  THIS AFFORIS
THE RECEIVING COUNTRY THE OPPORTUNITY TO EVALUATE THE
PROPOSED IMPORT AND TO REQUEST FURTHER INFORMATION CON-
CERNING THE WASTE AND TAKE APPROPRIATE ACTION IF IT SO
DESIRES.
```

This 1981 State Department dispatch concerns a plan of a company called Ashvins USA Inc. of Birmingham, Alabama, the officers of which include an Alabama state senator, Earl Goodwin, and a former Alabama state highway superintendent, Ray Bass, to export "toxic wastes to Bahamas."

GRAVETT LEONARD L   05/11/81 164652   PRINTER: FF
81 STATE 1522

LIMITED OFFICIAL USE   **DECLASSIFIED**   F. Earl
PAGE 01   STATE   001522
ORIGIN OES-09
INFO OCT-00   AF-10   ARA-12   ADS-00   AID-07   CEQ-01   CIAE-00
      H-01   COME-00 DODE-00 EB-08   EPA-01   INR-10   IO-14
      L-03   NSF-01   NSC-05   NSAE-00 PM-07   ICA-11   SS-15
      SP-02   DOE-10   INT-05   ACDA-12 SPRS-02 SMI-01   DLOS-05
      CG-00   DOTE-30   /136 R
DRAFTED BY OES/ENH:SPATTERSON
APPROVED BY OES/ENH:DBLACK
EB:GJOHNSON (INFO)
EPA/OIA:CSASTIAN (INFO)
ARA/CAR:KMCINTYRE (INFO)
S/P:BECKHOLM (INFO)
OES/E:MHOINKES

P 030702Z JAN 81
FM SECSTATE WASHDC
TO AMEMBASSY NASSAU
INFO AMEMBASSY GUATEMALA
AMEMBASSY TEGUCIGALPA
AMCONSUL CAPE TOWN
LIMITED OFFICIAL USE STATE 001522
E.O. 12065: N/A
AGS:SENV
SUBJECT: PROPOSED EXPORT OF TOXIC WASTES TO BAHAMAS
SUMMARY: ALABAMA FIRM ASHVINS USA IS CONSIDERING EXPORT
OF HAZARDOUS WASTES TO CARNARVON LTD., NASSAU, BAHAMAS.
ASHVINS HAS CONTACTED DEPT. REGARDING PROPOSED ARRANGEMENT.
DEPT. HAS ADVISED GOB AMB. WOODS OF MATTER. EMBASSY'S
VIEWS AND ANY INFORMATION EMBASSY MAY HAVE ON MATTER ARE
LIMITED OFFICIAL USE
LIMITED OFFICIAL USE
PAGE 02   STATE   001522
REQUESTED. END SUMMARY.
2. DEPT. WAS VISITED BY TWO REPRESENTATIVES OF ASHVINS
USA INC. OF BIRMINGHAM, ALABAMA, ONE A LOCAL ATTORNEY AND
THE OTHER ALABAMA STATE SENATOR EARL GOODWIN FROM SELMA.
THE FIRM HAS ENTERED INTO NEGOTIATIONS WITH LAWRENCE G.
CHISHOLM, CARNARVON LTD., 42 QUEEN ST., NASSAU, REGARDING
SHIPMENT OF US ORIGIN TOXIC WASTES TO CARNARVON'S WASTE
DISPOSAL FACILITY IN THE BAHAMAS. ASHVINS LETTER TO
CARNARVON STATES QUOTE WE WOULD DELIVER TO YOU, ON BARGES,
WASTE MATERIALS EACH MONTH. WHEN THE BARGE ARRIVES AT
YOUR DESIGNATED SITE, IT SHALL CONTAIN 8,800 BARRELS OF
WASTE UNQUOTE. CARNARVON WOULD UNLOAD, STORE OR DISPOSE
OF THE MATERIALS. ASHVINS WOULD BE GRANTED EXCLUSIVE
RIGHT FOR BUSINESS WITH THE US. REPORTEDLY THE ATTORNEY
GENERAL OF THE BAHAMAS IS SENDING ASHVINS A LETTER
APPROVING THE ARRANGEMENT, AND ASHVINS WILL SUPPLY DEPT.
WITH A COPY WHICH WE WILL TRANSMIT TO
LIMITED OFFICIAL USE /

GRAVETT LEONARD L   05/11/81 164654   PRINTER: FF
31 STATE 1522
DECLASSIFIED USE
EMBASSY.
3. ASHVINS INTENDS TO GATHER WASTE MATERIALS FROM 8-
STATE REGION, AND STORE THEM AT SEVERAL SITES UNTIL
SHIPMENT. ALTHOUGH ASHVINS CLAIMS TO HAVE AN INTERIM
LICENSE ISSUED BY EPA'S REGIONAL OFFICE IN ATLANTA, ACCORD
-ING TO THAT OFFICE THE ISSUE IS STILL PENDING. AMONG
THE WASTES CONTEMPLATED FOR EXPORT ARE PCB'S WHICH MUST
BE INCINERATED AT HIGH TEMPERATURES AND UNDER CAREFUL
CONDITIONS FOR SAFE DISPOSAL. ASHVINS STATES THAT A
PROPOSED INCINERATOR ADEQUATE TO HANDLE PCB'S WILL BE
CONSTRUCTED IN THE BAHAMAS, AND IN THE MEANTIME, OTHER
WASTE DISPOSAL WILL BEGIN.
LIMITED OFFICIAL USE
LIMITED OFFICIAL USE
PAGE 03   STATE 001522
4. NEW US REGULATIONS GOVERNING WASTES "FROM CRADLE TO
GRAVE" UNDER THE RESOURCE CONSERVATION AND RECOVERY ACT
WENT INTO EFFECT NOVEMBER 19. THESE REGULATIONS, WHICH
MAY MAKE LEGAL DISPOSAL OF WASTES IN THE US MORE COSTLY,
MAY THEREFORE CREATE AN INCREASED INCENTIVE TO EXPORT.
ASHVINS WAS INCORPORATED NOVEMBER 13, AND ITS ENTIRE
OPERATION IS DIRECTED TO THE EXPORT OF WASTES. THE
COMPANY REPORTEDLY IS IN PRELIMINARY NEGOTIATIONS IN
HONDURAS AND GUATEMALA AS WELL, AND POSSIBLY WITH OTHER
CARIBBEAN OR CENTRAL AMERICAN COUNTRIES.

Ashvins' promotional literature tells prospective customers: "Unlike landfill sites in the United States where the generators' waste is identified as to source and made part of the burial records for perpetuity, Ashvins . . . submits export documents without generator identification to the foreign company . . . While it is known what substances are handled, it is not known where it was generated. This method holds the generator's name in confidence and eliminates any liability in the years to come."

Bass, treasurer of Ashvins, said the plan involved "a wonderful idea because it's an acceptable method of removing waste from this country . . . It's much safer than your Love Canals and Valley of the Drums."

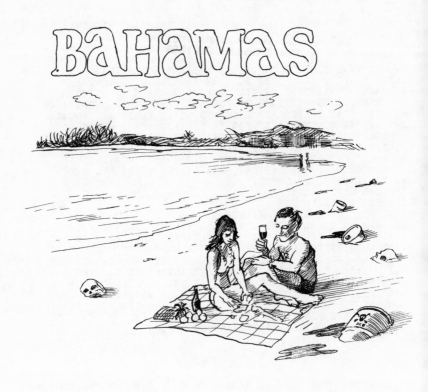

And while some U.S. corporations are preparing to use nations around the world as dumping grounds for toxic wastes from America, other U.S. companies are principals in a multi-billion dollar toxic chemical trade which includes the peddling globally of millions of pounds of toxic pesticides—including some so dangerous that they wouldn't even be allowed to be used in America under the EPA's weak standards.

This is a key to the 500,000 pesticide poisonings worldwide every year—a pesticide poisoning every minute!—as estimated by the World Health Organization, and to the deaths of 22,500 persons annually from pesticides, as estimated by the Britain-based Oxford Committee on Famine Relief.

DDT, aldrin, Parathion, Kepone—among other deadly pesticides—may have finally become outlawed or had their use restricted in the U.S., but that doesn't stop American companies from peddling these and other toxic substances to other nations, particularly Third World countries where environmental laws are virtually nonexistent.

There have been several journalistic exposés on the issue of America's international traffic in toxic chemicals.

But still, the situation has just become worse—because of the huge power of the poison traffickers and their grip on the U.S. government.

Newsweek in 1981 did a report on "Pesticides' Global Fallout." It started with this description:

"Farmers in the Phillipines regularly spray their fields with Parathion, a highly toxic pesticide. Unaware of the chemical's harmful effects, three rural tribesman once turned hoses on each other as a joke. They all died. A farm-supply store in Haiti is packed with multicolored drums of pesticides—many of them banned in the United States. Clerks scoop out the toxic white powders with their bare hands and put them into unlabeled plastic bags for sale to farmers to use on their crops. When the drums are empty, they are sold, unwashed, to peasants who use them as water containers."

And it included the declaration of Jack Early, president of the National Agricultural Chemicals Association, "We should not impose on these countries a standard that we have imposed on ourselves."

Bob Wyrick, in a 1981 investigative report for *Newsday* entitled "Hazards for Export," wrote of "patterns of exploitation that often victimize the consumer, endanger the worker and poison the environment. The practices often involve actions that would be prohibited at home, such as exposing employees to unsafe working conditions and promoting and selling goods that have been judged too hazardous for the domestic market." American business executives interviewed "saw no need to defend themselves." The White House deputy adviser for consumer affairs said: "We can't be the world's nanny."

A 1981 Public Broadcasting Service report, on "Pesticides and Pills, For Export Only," began with the scene in

Achedemade Bator, a small village in Ghana, where fish from Lake Volta is the main source of food. Said the narrator: "Fishermen from Achedemade Bator showed us how they used to catch fish. They did it by poisoning them with a chemical called Gammalin 20. The fishermen poured it into the lake water, which is also their only source of drinking water. They got the chemical from women who bought small bottles or cans of it in local shops and came to the village to trade for fish. In the United States, Gammalin 20 is called Lindane. Hooker Chemical, a subsidiary of Occidental Petroleum, produces it." Lindane has been restricted in the U.S. and Europe since 1969, but in this West African nation it can be purchased like Coca-Cola. Meanwhile, "the fishermen of Achedemade Bator noticed about a ten percent decline in the number and size of the fish they caught in each of several years. Without fish the village cannot survive."

"This film is about double standards," the documentary began. "It is about certain pesticides and medications we in the United States and other industrial nations export to developing countries in the Third World, products totally banned or severely restricted." These are "products known to cause cancer and birth deformities in animals, to cause blood disorders, paralysis, blindness, sterility, even death among people."

With great irony much of the pesticide-laced food from overseas, including produce doused with poisons regarded as too toxic for spraying in the U.S., return to America on imported food.

In 1979, the General Accounting Office issued this report on the U.S. poison boomerang:

BY THE COMPTROLLER GENERAL

Report To The Congress
OF THE UNITED STATES

Better Regulation Of Pesticide Exports And Pesticide Residues In Imported Food Is Essential

Pesticides suspended, canceled, or never registered for use in the United States because of hazards associated with their use are exported routinely. Serious injuries have occurred from the use of these pesticides in other countries. The Environmental Protection Agency in many cases has neither informed other governments of pesticide suspensions, cancellations, and restrictions in the United States nor revoked tolerances for residues of these pesticides on imported food.

The Food and Drug Administration does not analyze imported food for many potential residues. It allows food to be marketed before testing it for illegal residues. Importers are not penalized if their imports later are determined to contain illegal residues. The safety and appropriateness of some residues allowed on imported food has not been determined.

CED-79-43
JUNE 22, 1979

The report noted:

Each year the United States exports millions of pounds
of pesticides to foreign countries. A large portion of these
exports are pesticides that have been suspended or canceled
for U.S. use because they may cause cancer or otherwise endanger humans, wildlife, or the environment. The majority
of unregistered pesticides exported, however, involve products whose chemical contents are unknown and/or whose human
and environmental hazards have not been adequately evaluated.

The production and distribution of pesticides produced
solely for export are largely uncontrolled. Neither EPA nor
any other Federal agency monitors the content, destination,
and intended uses of such pesticides. Some exported pesticides have caused serious deaths and injuries in foreign
countries. In addition, exported pesticides that are used on
food crops in foreign countries, may be present as residues
on U.S. food imports. The extent to which imported food contains residues of harmful pesticides or pesticides whose hazards have not been adequately evaluated is unknown.

MAGNITUDE OF PESTICIDE EXPORTS

The Bureau of the Census reported that in calendar year
1976 over 552 million pounds of pesticides were exported from
the United States. (See app. III.) Available data shows
that over 161 million pounds, or 29 percent, represented
pesticides not registered for U.S. use. About 20 percent
of these unregistered pesticides--some 31 million pounds--
involve pesticides that EPA had suspended or canceled because
their uses posed unreasonable hazards to human life, wildlife, or the environment. A more significant portion of pesticide exports--some 130 million pounds--consists of products
that may never have been registered with EPA. Some unregistered pesticide exports consist of chemicals whose properties
have not been studied or, if studied, are considered too hazardous for U.S. use. Other unregistered pesticide products
may consist of "active ingredients" contained in registered
products, that differ from registered products only in their
formulations; that is the combinations and relative amounts
of active ingredients.

Nonetheless, EPA knows little about most of these
products and some undoubtedly contain chemicals that EPA has
not evaluated adequately for potential adverse effects.

*The production and distribution of pesticides produced
solely for export are largely uncontrolled.*

The report went on:

IMPORTED FOOD IS NOT TESTED FOR MANY

POTENTIALLY UNSAFE PESTICIDE RESIDUES

U.S. food imports may contain unsafe pesticide residues
because:

--Foreign nations permit use of pesticides which EPA
either does not permit or has not evaluated for
consumer safety.

--FDA's generally used multiresidue analysis tests
detect neither the bulk of pesticides with U.S. tolerances nor other pesticides never registered by the
United States which foreign nations use on food crops.

--FDA does not always identify unknown residues it de-
tects on imported food.

--FDA does not sample all significant food commodity imports for pesticide residues.

And it included this chart of specific foods sent into the
U.S., the exporting countries and the numbers of pesticides
involved:

Pesticides Used in Foreign Countries
on Food Exported to the United States

| Commodity | Countries surveyed | Number of pesticides | | |
		Allowed, recommended, or used	Having no U.S. tolerance	Not detectable with FDA tests
Bananas	Colombia, Costa Rica, Ecuador, Guatemala, Mexico	45	25	37
Coffee	Brazil, Colombia, Costa Rica, Ecuador, Guatemala, Mexico	94	76	64
Sugar	Brazil, Colombia, Costa Rica, Ecuador, Guatemala, India, Thailand	61	34	33
Tomatoes	Mexico, Spain	53	21	28
Tea	India, Sri Lanka	24	20	11
Cacao	Costa Rica, Ecuador	14	7	7
Tapioca	Thailand	4	4	1
Straw-berries	Mexico	13	-	5
Peppers	Mexico	12	-	4
Olives	Italy, Spain	20	14	8

The report stressed:

In some countries, hazardous pesticides are used extensively.

--Brazil, Ecuador, and other major Central American banana-producing countries apply benomyl--a pesticide suspected of causing cancer, birth defects, and gene mutations--to bananas 12 to 20 times annually.

--An estimated one-fifth of the world's parathion is applied in the small nation of El Salvador--sixth largest source of U.S. coffee imports.

--In Nicaragua, Honduras, Guatemala, and El Salvador use of DDT, dieldrin, toxaphene, endrin, and methyl and ethyl parathion on cotton has contaminated food, feed, water, and wildlife. For example, Guatemalan milk was found to be contaminated with DDT residues at levels 90 times the U.S. tolerance. Over seven percent of all U.S. agricultural imports originate in these four countries.

It provided this chart:

Food on Which Foreign Countries Allow Use
of Suspended and Canceled Pesticides

Pesticide	Country			
	Ecuador	Guatemala	Costa Rica	India
Aldrin	cacao coffee	coffee sugar	coffee	sugar tea
Dieldrin	coffee	bananas sugar coffee	bananas coffee cacao	
Heptachlor		sugar	sugar cacao	sugar
Chlordane	cacao		coffee	
DDT		bananas		
Kepone		bananas		

And it concluded:

COMPTROLLER GENERAL'S REPORT TO THE CONGRESS	BETTER REGULATION OF PESTICIDE EXPORTS AND PESTICIDE RESIDUES IN IMPORTED FOOD IS ESSENTIAL

D I G E S T

World demand for pesticides is growing. Developing countries are expected to become more and more dependent on pesticides as they improve food and fiber production. For example, the dollar value of Africa's pesticide demand is expected to increase more than fivefold during the decade ending in 1984.

American agricultural imports in fiscal year 1977 totaled over $13 <u>billion</u>, making other countries' pesticide practices increasingly important because pesticide residues may be on these imports. The Food and Drug Administration--whose job is to assure that marketed food is safe, pure, and wholesome--has identified neither the pesticide practices of nor all pesticides used in other countries. Such knowledge is essential if the agency is to make sure that food imports do not contain harmful residues of pesticides that have been suspended, canceled, or never registered in the United States.

CONCLUSIONS

Imported food may be contaminated with pesticides not allowed in the United States or with pesticide residues in excess of legally established U.S. limits. Many pesticides permitted in foreign countries have no U.S. tolerances.

FDA does not know what pesticide residues may be present in imported food because neither FDA nor Department of State officials gather data on overseas pesticide use. Lacking knowledge of likely residues, FDA is unable to effectively determine which tests should be conducted on imported food to ensure its safety and purity.

In 1980, Representative Michael Barnes of Maryland introduced a bill which would restrict the export of hazardous products from the U.S.

It has gotten nowhere.

In one of his last acts as president, Jimmy Carter—after waffling on the issue because of industry pressure, admitted The White House—issued an executive order toughening notification requirements when a company wants to export a product whose use is restricted in the U.S.

In one of his first acts as president, Ronald Reagan revoked the month-old Carter order and his administration has drafted guidelines that water down or eliminate what few rules exist on exporting U.S. poison.

The administration proposes to "eliminate certain requirements for providing notice of specific exports to recipient countries" because "in the past such notices have placed U.S. exports at a competitive disadvantage."

America can now expand its program of poisoning the world.

Asks Jacob Scherr, an attorney for the Natural Resources Defense Council: "Do we have a license to misrepresent, to maim and kill people overseas?"

And as David Weir and Mark Schapiro wrote in their 1981 book published by the San Francisco-based Institute for Food and Development Policy, it's literally a *Circle of Poison*.

"We are victims, too," they stressed. "Pesticide exports create a circle of poison, disabling workers in American chemical plants and later returning to us in the food we import. Drinking a morning coffee or enjoying a luncheon salad, the American consumer is eating pesticides banned or restricted in the United States, but legally shipped to the Third World."

What is involved is "chemical colonialism" they declared. "A few executives from a handful of multinational corporations and their government allies are allowed to make decisions affecting entire peoples."

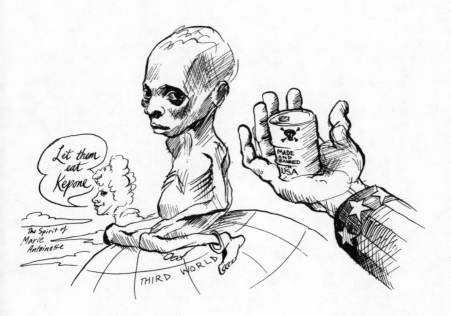

Cornucopia

"We propose a 'people's conspiracy' which we call The Cornucopia Project," declared Robert Rodale in 1980.

"The Cornucopia Project is three things," says Rodale, editor of the Rodale Press, publishers of *Organic Gardening, Prevention* and other magazines stressing natural farming and living. "First, it is a collection of technical information about the U.S. food system that people can use to plan new ways to fight the food-cost inflation that is an ever-increasing problem. Second, The Cornucopia Project is an effort to structure the food system in ways that will make organic growing more practical, thus helping to create a truly sustainable and permanent way of producing food. Finally, it is a potentially valuable planning tool for farmers and those food companies—especially the smaller ones—that have an interest in using organic techniques."

Based in Emmaus, Pennsylvania, the home of the Rodale Press, The Cornucopia Project has attracted many thousands of members, now has a full staff, and has been busily analyzing and helping others analyze the U.S. food system all with the aim of changing the system's recent directions and sending it on safe, non-poisonous, more economical, more fruitful paths.

221

Among the issues explored by The Cornucopia Project in its report, *Organic Paths to Food Security,* were:

Food quality. Increased crop yields have not led to any increase in food quality. Chemical bombardment starts with the seed and ends only when the food is finally packaged. And these alien substances remain to pollute our environment and our bodies.

The swing toward more processed foods has also contributed to nutritional problems. Heart disease can be partly attributed to excess saturated fat and refined carbohydrates in the diet. Lack of fiber is strongly suspected of promoting certain kinds of cancer. Increased consumption of sugar has led to more tooth decay. All the evidence points in one direction: the further our system has strayed from fresh, simple food, the more health problems we have had.

Pollution. The increasing use of herbicides, pesticides, and chemical fertilizers has led to the contamination of our soil and water, and the destruction of wildlife. The environmental impact of these substances costs an estimated $839 million annually. And this does not include any damage that may result as these chemicals concentrate up the food chain and find their way into our bodies.

Increased pesticide use also tends to encourage the development of stronger pests, which in turn leads to more powerful pesticides. Already, to grow our crops, we use approximately 6¼ pounds of pesticide for every person in the country.

Fertilizer use. Our high production levels are dependent on chemical fertilizers, especially those that supply the three essential plant nutrients—phosphorus, nitrogen, and potassium. We now use an average of 120 pounds of synthetic fertilizer nutrients per acre of cropland each year, which amounts to more than 200 pounds for every person in the country. Without this fertilizer, yields would drop an estimated 30 to 40 percent.

Yet our supplies of these products are tenuous. We are currently running out of phosphate rock—our reserves are expected to be gone shortly after 2000—but we continue to export about one-fourth of our production. We already produce less than half of the potassium (in the form of potash) we need, and projections are that in 20 years we will produce only 10 percent of the required amount. We can get all the nitrogen we need from the air, but it requires so much natural gas to process it into a usable form (usually ammonia) that the cost is rising astronomically. And when our natural gas supplies run out and we have to switch to making ammonia with new technologies, the cost will go even higher.

The Cornucopia Project sets these goals for a food system:

Abundant. The food system should produce enough so that everyone's nutritional needs are met. This should also include a good quality and choice of foods.

Safe. All food should be grown, processed, and distributed in a way that is as safe as possible for workers, for the environment, and for those who eat the food.

Efficient. The food system should use less energy, and move as far as possible toward use of renewable energy.

Appropriate. The food system should be flexible enough to meet various local needs, and each region should work for as much self-sufficiency as practical.

Participatory. The food system should be open so that there is maximum opportunity for individuals to be involved in the decisions made at every level.

Changeable. The food system should welcome change and growth, and be flexible enough to adapt in times of stress or disaster.

A "sustainable" food system is the "overall aim," a system not dependent on "rapidly disappearing fossil fuels or chemical fertilizers; it should preserve our soil from erosion and our environment from pollution. It should be a food system that can be sustained indefinitely, and provide for the food needs of our children and grandchildren."

And "to realize these goals, many important changes would have to be made in our food system" including farmers moving "from conventional, chemical farming techniques to more sustainable, organic methods that conserve both soil and energy," and more food should be grown "at home and in our local communities."

Rodale says: "Looking at our food system, we need to switch it away from being a mining operation. We are mining the soil of its fertility, and are draining oil and gas fields of their wealth to get the energy to do that. Mines always run out and become depleted. We can't afford to let our food system just 'run out' someday.

"Widespread application of organic farming techniques is the way to build permanence into our farms. Organic farming feeds the soil instead of mining it. Humus is built up, creating an intensely alive soil environment that liberates minerals and other nutrients gradually in ways that allow a soil to remain fertile for many thousands of years. There is also recycling of nutrients. Rotations which include legumes both capture nitrogen from the air and help to prevent erosion. Pollution of soil, water, air and food is prevented because toxic chemicals are not used."

"Mother Nature Bats Last," was the title of a 1981 article by Rodale in *Organic Gardening* in which he stressed that "it's time we stop trying to play tricks on Mother Nature, and realize that the human environment that we must create for ourselves will work only as long as the natural environment retains its fundamental integrity. In effect, we are in a game, and . . . Mother Nature bats last. We can 'load the bases' with new technologies, and even hit a bunch of home runs. But somewhere out there is another player, whom we can't see, who is always going to come to the plate."

Out of Raytown, Missouri, Charles Walters, Jr. has articulated a similar message through *Acres, U.S.A.* which emphasizes it is *A Voice For Eco-Agriculture*. On the masthead is also the line, "To Be Economical, Agriculture Has To Be Ecological."

Walters began the newspaper 11 years ago.

"It became transparently obvious that the technological advice to farmers was at least as bad as the economic advice," he is saying, so he became publisher and editor of a now thick, natural farming-oriented newspaper.

He says: "There is a little story about a young fellow in the

early Christian era. He found Christians being fed to the lions, and other unhappy things, so he hid in the desert. The Lord came to him and asked, 'Why are you hiding?' The young fellow related the situation in Rome, and said he believed Christians would all be wiped out. For this reason, he hid in the desert—to save the Word. The Lord said, 'Go back to Rome and preach the doctrine. Someone will hear. And you need not worry about being wrong or taking the blame for anything. Because when the Word is passed along, it will be someone else's idea. The ideas we have in *Acres U.S.A.* all belong to others—now, in the past, and in the future."
And they are the soundest of concepts.

Walters wrote in the editorial in the first issue that for "too long, the thinking and ideas that affect the topsoil of our nation have come from pedants and industrial practioners who keep looking for a fast buck at the expense of posterity . . . our exploitative type of agricultural production is a disgrace and must be corrected quickly."

An editorial in 1981 on "The Real Danger Facing America" declared that the "intellectual advisors to the farmer have counseled toxic technology, namely simplistic salt fertilizers and toxic rescue chemistry. Those hooked on this chemical fix cannot farm any other way. They have forgotten almost everything they ever knew about nature and rely chiefly on reading the labels on cans and packages. Their soil systems are on the fix much like a narcotics addict, and in almost all cases the organic matter and humus supply has been wasted away to a point where a comeback will require a long and disciplined regimen of rejuvenation.

"The predictions are not hard to make, and they are not hard to keep accurate. Not understood as well is how the American public will react to its cup of hemlock. Mental acuity has been sinking with each step in the debasement of food supply, and it is almost impossible at this point to measure the damage. In the past, Americans have bounced back when faced with adversity, but this was before the chemical industry had zapped the population."

Natural farming practices are not just the subject of words and wishes.

They are being practiced actively, widely and successfully.

Despite "the great American agribusiness myth, chemical farming is not the only way. Organic farming works," noted Daniel Zwerdling in a 1978 report in *New Times*. "During an investigation that took me from the Corn Belt to the fertile farms of Europe, I found large-scale, sophisticated, commercial farms raising high-quality foods organically—lush citrus orchards and vast acres of cauliflower and broccoli and peppers and soft lettuce. I found scientific studies conducted by major research centers in Europe—studies virtually ignored in the United States—which suggest that organically grown foods can be not only as good as their chemical counterparts but in some ways superior.

"And while I had always assumed that farmers go organic to earn spiritual points while conventional farmers go the chemical route to earn money, here's the biggest irony: The organic farmers I spoke with have abandoned their chemical habits in the past decade precisely because the financial and ecological costs of the chemical system were driving them out of business."

Studies have shown that the net dollar return per acre for organic and chemical farmers is virtually the same. One such study was conducted between 1974 and 1976 by the Center for Biology of Natural Systems at Washington University in St. Louis. Fourteen organic farms—up to 800 acres in size—located in Illinois, Iowa, Minnesota, Nebraska and Missouri were each compared with "nearby conventionally operated" farms which used chemicals and were reputed to be highly successful. A generally slightly higher crop yield—of 10%—was found in the conventional farms and that was made up for by the organic farmers having lower costs.

The chemical industry is extremely concerned about the threat posed to it by non-toxic, natural farming and with its many allies in government tries to discourage such agriculture. As former U.S. Agriculture Secretary Earl Butz proclaimed on national television: "Before we go back to organic agriculture in this country, somebody must decide which 50 million Americans we are going to let starve or go hungry."

But somehow, this thoroughly positive report on organic farming got through the apparatus and was issued by the U.S. government in 1980:

REPORT AND RECOMMENDATIONS ON ORGANIC FARMING

 UNITED STATES DEPARTMENT OF AGRICULTURE

Organic farming was defined by the Department of Agriculture team as "a production system which avoids or largely excludes the use of synthetically compounded fertilizers, pesticides, growth regulators, and livestock feed additives. To the maximum extent feasible, organic farming systems rely upon crop rotations, crop residues, animal manures, legumes, green manures, off-farm organic wastes, mechanical cultivation, mineral-bearing rocks, and aspects of biological pest control to maintain soil productivity and tilth, to supply plant nutrients, and to control insects, weeds, and other pests."

And the principal findings of the study were these points:

- Organic farming operations are not limited by scale. This study found that while there are many small-scale (10 to 50 acres) organic farmers in the northeastern region, there are a significant number of large-scale (more than 100 acres and even up to 1,500 acres) organic farms in the West and Midwest. In most cases, the team members found that these farms, both large and small, were productive, efficient, and well managed.
- Motivations for shifting from chemical farming to organic farming include concern for protecting soil, human, and animal health from the potential hazards of pesticides; the desire for lower production inputs; concern for the environment and protection of soil resources.
- Contrary to popular belief, most organic farmers have not regressed to agriculture as it was practiced in the 1930's. While they attempt to avoid or restrict the use of chemical fertilizers and pesticides, organic farmers still use modern farm machinery, recommended crop varieties, certified seed, sound methods of organic waste management, and recommended soil and water conservation practices.
- Most organic farmers use crop rotations that include legumes and cover crops to provide an adequate supply of nitrogen for moderate to high yields.
- Animals comprise an essential part of the operation of many organic farms. In a mixed crop/livestock operation, grains and forages are fed on the farm and the manure is returned to the land. Sometimes the manure is composted to conserve nitrogen, and in some cases farmers import both feed and manure from off-farm sources.
- The study team was impressed by the ability of organic farmers to control weeds in crops such as corn, soybeans, and cereals without the use (or with only minimal use) of herbicides. Their success here is attributed to timely tillage and cultivation, delayed planting, and crop rotations. They have also been relatively successful in controlling insect pests.

- Some organic farmers expressed the feeling that they have been neglected by the U.S. Department of Agriculture and the land-grant universities. They believe that both Extension agents and researchers, for the most part, have little interest in organic methods and that they have no one to turn to for help on technical problems.

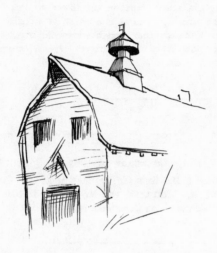

The report concluded, "Moreover, many organic farmers have developed unique and innovative methods of organic recycling and pest control in their crop production sequences. Because of these and other reasons outlined in this report, the team feels strongly that research and education programs should be developed to address the needs and problems of organic farmers. Certainly, much can be learned from a holistic research effort to investigate the organic system of farming, its mechanisms, interactions, principles, and potential benefits to agriculture both at home and abroad."

Introduced and moving uphill very slowly in Congress since the government report on organic farming is the Organic Farming Act of 1982. Here it is:

97TH CONGRESS
2D SESSION
H. R. 5618

To require the Secretary of Agriculture to establish a network of volunteers to
assist in making available information and advice on organic agriculture for
family farms and other agricultural enterprises, to establish pilot projects to
carry out research and education activities involving organic farming, and to
perform certain other functions relating to organic farming, with special
emphasis on family farms.

IN THE HOUSE OF REPRESENTATIVES

FEBRUARY 24, 1982

Mr. WEAVER (for himself, Mr. BEDELL, Mr. DASCHLE, Mr. VENTO, Mr. SABO,
Mr. GEJDENSON, Ms. MIKULSKI, and Mr. NEAL) introduced the following
bill; which was referred to the Committee on Agriculture

A BILL

To require the Secretary of Agriculture to establish a network
of volunteers to assist in making available information and
advice on organic agriculture for family farms and other
agricultural enterprises, to establish pilot projects to carry
out research and education activities involving organic farming, and to perform certain other functions relating to organic farming, with special emphasis on family farms.

1   *Be it enacted by the Senate and House of Representa-*
2 *tives of the United States of America in Congress assembled,*

It was introduced by Representative Jim Weaver of Oregon in the House, Vermont's Senator Patrick Leahy in the Senate.

The Department of Agriculture, interestingly, has been the prime opponent of the bill.

Since its introduction, the wording for the "purpose" of the act has been changed from "to facilitate and promote the scientific investigation and understanding of methods of organic farming and to assist farmers and other producers to use methods of organic farming to *replace* conventional chemical-intensive methods of farming" to "*complement* conventional chemical-intensive methods of farming."

Says Weaver: "Many farmers lack information on alternative agricultural systems. They are understandably hesitant to make a transition because any change entails a certain amount of economic risk. This is especially true today, with the tremendous economic pressures facing most family farmers. There is a great need for practical demonstrations and proven research to help farmers make this transition to what promises to be a more efficient, economic and substainable form of agriculture."

Cornucopia lies ahead, although the Poison Conspiracy would keep it hidden.

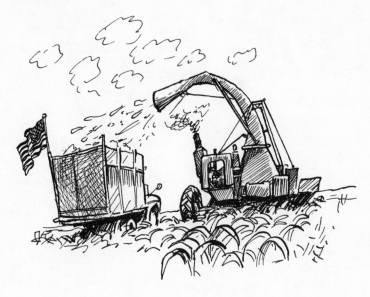

Conclusion

It was all very well to say "Drink me," but the wise little Alice was not going to do *that* in a hurry; "No, I'll look first," she said, "and see whether it's marked *'poison'* or not"; for she had read several nice little stories about children who had got burnt, and eaten up by wild beasts, and other unpleasant things, all because they *would* not remember the simple rules their friends had taught them, such as, that a red-hot poker will burn you if you hold it too long; and that, if you cut your finger *very* deeply with a knife it usually bleeds; and she had never forgotten that if you drink very much from a bottle marked "poison," it is almost certain to disagree with you, sooner or later.

—*Alice in Wonderland*

We are people in poisonland.

In *Silent Spring* in 1962 Rachel Carson wrote: "For the first time in the history of the world, every human being is now subjected to contact with dangerous chemicals."

Twenty years later, the situation has grown worse—and can be expected to worsen further. Because the incubation or latency period is usually decades before poisons manifest themselves as cancer, the full harvest of illness and death is yet to arrive. And as toxins continue to be spread throughout the environment in larger and larger volumes, by the time the scale of the tragedy ahead is realized, it could easily be too late. The curve of death is still far from peaking.

An awareness of what has been happening has led to passage of some laws.

233

As the Council on Environmental Quality noted in its 1977 annual report:

> But the major accomplishment of the new law is that it gives the government broad authority to control the production, distribution, and use of *all* potentially hazardous chemicals. It provides for testing of suspect chemicals before they become widely used and economically important. It emphasizes collection of information and freedom of access to research data so that the scientific community can note and assess potential problems.
>
> Although we now have most of the basic legal tools for the task, it will not be accomplished easily. It will require coordination of research and regulation by many agencies under a dozen or more major federal laws, a program to fill information gaps and provide easy access to the data that exist, adequate funding, and intensive effort by trained people.

Until the Toxic Substances Control Act of 1976 was passed, there was simply no way to assess or control the development, production, and marketing of the flood of manmade chemicals. Many of these complex chemicals do a great deal of good and little harm, but some are among the most toxic and persistent substances ever introduced into our environment.

Unhappily, the toxicity and persistence of chemicals have often been discovered *after* their widespread use and *after* they have become important to jobs, commerce, or agriculture.

Although perhaps we now have "the basic legal tools for the task," there is not the will, not the commitment to do the job.

"We're treating more acres and using more pesticides than ever before," says David Pimentel, professor of entomology and agricultural sciences at Cornell University. "Even after Rachel Carson, we haven't gained a whole lot."

"Agriculture goes on being increasingly chemicalized," says Boisie E. Day, professor emeritus of plant physiology at the University of California at Berkeley.

Production of pesticides has doubled in the United States

since *Silent Spring*—from 730 million pounds in 1962 to almost 1.5 billion pounds in 1980.

Indeed, more and more chemical pesticides are needed as insects become resistant; some 400 insect species are now resistant to one or more pesticides, at latest count. And pest damage is twice as bad as it was before chemical pesticides were invented.

The chemical companies, meanwhile, aggressively concoct other poisons, churn them out and spend millions upon millions creating and holding markets for the toxins.

As a Hooker Chemicals' bulletin explains: "The research department is free to develop any product that looks promising. If there is not a market for it, the sales development group seeks to create one."

Toxic waste dumping continues unbridled.

"On the 20th anniversary of *Silent Spring,* pesticides and other deadly chemicals remain a greater threat than ever. We're in the midst of a cancer epidemic, a lot of it associated with toxic chemicals," says Lewis Regenstein, author of *America the Poisoned* and vice president of Fund for Animals.

The National Cancer Institute in 1981 issued a report increasing the number of Americans it projects as getting cancer in their lifetimes—up to one in three, and one in six will die from it, it said.

New research comes out such as the 1982 study by the University of Medicine and Dentistry of New Jersey which found that the death rate from three types of cancer in the highly-industrialized and contaminated northeastern corridor of New Jersey exceeded the national average by 50%. "I think somehow people don't realize that if you want to face the major problem for this country over the next 20 years, it's the disposal of hazardous wastes," says Donald B. Louria, the chairman of the university's department of preventive medicine and community health. "I don't think the American public is nearly as concerned and constructively aggressive as it should be."

But the public has been pounded down by the poisoners.

One would think the poisoners would understand that it is "their soup," too.

I interviewed a former public relations person for American Cyanamid on this point. He asked that his name not be published because "I have a lot of friends still there." The ex-PR man recounted: "When I started at American Cyanamid I was handed a copy of Rachel Carson's *Silent Spring,* and I was told your first assignment will be rebutting this; eliminate her." American Cyanamid then and now has specialized in selling pesticides based on formulas developed by the Nazis for nerve gas during World War II, organophosphates which are not as persistent as the chlorinated hydrocarbons Miss Carson emphasized in *Silent Spring.* "After reading the book, I went back to my boss," said the ex-PR man, "and said, 'Rachel Carson is doing a selling job for us. We don't make chlorinated hydrocarbons.' The answer to that was, 'No, the industry sticks together. Don't even think that way.'

"Never," said the ex-PR man, did American Cyanamid reflect on the charges. "The criticism was never taken seriously," he said. "Did we try to clean up our act? Absolutely not!"

In his years at American Cyanamid, he said he found "not a scintilla" of thinking about "whether there's any truth in this. Instead, it was a total stonewall."

"The companies just don't give a shit about the public," he declared. Their sole concern is "having record profits and earnings every year."

As to their poisons coming back to injure or kill corporate executives or their families, "you can fool yourself to believe anything," said the ex-PR man, and the salaries and the positions of the corporate officials provide them with the incentive to fool themselves.

Denial is how the EPA ultimately handled Love Canal contamination, by simply announcing in 1982 that the area was again "habitable"—a claim met by wide disbelief.

An ultimate in corporate irresponsibility—and denial—also came in 1982 when the Manville Corporation handled 16,000 lawsuits stemming from the Manville's manufacture of cancer-causing asbestos by declaring bankruptcy despite its $2.3 billion in assets. Full-page newspaper advertisements were run in which the company's president and chief executive officer, John A. McKinney, outlined Manville's strategy:

Manville

For further information write to the Corporate Relations Department, Manville Corporation,
P.O. Box 5108, Denver Colorado 80217

Q. Mr. McKinney, this announcement was a surprise. What's wrong with Manville's operations?
A. *Nothing is wrong with our businesses. Filing Chapter 11 does not mean that the Company is going out of business or that its assets will be liquidated. Thousands of asbestos-health lawsuits are the problem!* We're the American and world leader in a number of markets, mostly related to construction. During the current recession our sales have held up well and we've operated at better than break even (if you exclude litigation expenses). We've slimmed down too, having eliminated more than 1500 salaried jobs in the last six months. We'll continue to generate substantial cash flow. Our Chapter 11 lawyers tell me Manville has stronger businesses and cash flow than any other big company that's ever filed.

McKinney complained that the asbestos injury suits were projected as costing $40,000 a case. So rather than compensating the tens of thousands of people who received cancer from the poison sold by Manville, the company was declaring bankruptcy to shield itself. It was saying: consumers drop dead. And it planned to merrily keep on with business as usual.

"It's a fairly ruthless act by Manville to escape liability to a lot of injured and diseased workers they have responsibility for," commented Representative George Miller of California.

"It's outrageous that a company would use the legal process to deny us our day in court," said Mary Trerotola of Harrison, New York, the widow of a victim of asbestos. But the purveyors of poison have been using governmental processes for years to get away with what they have been doing.

And the courts are no exception.

The Poisoning of Michigan by Joyce Egginton is about how, in 1973, the Michigan Chemical Corporation, a subsidiary of the Velsicol Chemical Corporation, delivered bags of polybrominated biphenyl—PBB, similar to PCB's—to an agricultural feed company. It was mixed into cattle feed and delivered across the state. Soon whole herds were devastated by a plague. Ultimately, 30,000 cattle, 1.5 million chickens and 7,700 other farm animals had to be destroyed. Meanwhile, federal and state authorities ignored or minimized the situation. And during the nine months it took before one chemist-turned-farmer, working on his own, came upon the real cause and the many more months before all the animals were dealt with, contaminated meat, milk and eggs were sold throughout the state and its nine million residents were poisoned. The April 1982 issue of the *Journal of the American Medical Association* contained a report by researchers from the Mount Sinai School of Medicine in New York that 97% of Michigan's 9.2 million residents now have measurable amounts of the toxic poison in their tissues. Virtually all people who lived in Michigan in 1973–1974 became poisoned. Many have developed diseases since.

"The contamination of Michigan was probably the most widespread, and the least reported, chemical disaster ever to happen in the western world," noted Miss Egginton.

Government was derelict. At one point, FDA scientist Albert Kobye, Jr. told Michigan legislators that exposures of people in Michigan to PBB was "so insignificant that no further federal action is warranted." For state agencies, too, inaction was the rule in the hope, wrote Miss Egginton, that "if the problem was ignored it might disappear. Instead it spread and worsened" and she quotes one Michigan state legislator as saying, "They tried to sweep it under the rug, and they swept so hard it came out the other side."

And when the victims "turned in desperation to the courts," they were easily shot down by "the superior resources of those corporate giants . . . responsible for poisoning their bodies and their land."

The stories repeat and repeat: people and the environment are poisoned and government is in league with the poisoners.

ITEM: Dr. Melvin Reuber, head of the federal government's Experimental Pathology Laboratory at the Frederick Cancer Research Center in Maryland, is "forced to resign his post" in September 1981 for determining after research that the pesticide malathion is carcinogenic. He is forced out "after criticism by his superior for 'actions that negatively affected' the economy of agricultural and rural communities in California and Wisconsin," reports the *Los Angeles Times*.

ITEM: The regional attorney in New York City for the New York State Department of Environmental Conservation "has been suspended after complaining to officials that the agency had failed to halt pollution violations by the city." Samuel J. Kearing, Jr. says in an April 1982 interview "that he believed his suspension was the result of his contention that 'the City of New York is the worst polluter in this region,' " reports *The New York Times*.

ITEM: EPA officials—including Anne Gorsuch—are sued in Federal District Court in Tampa, Florida in March 1982 for having "failed to carry out environmental protection regulations." The EPA and the Army Corps of Engineers have been allowing the dumping of contaminated materials, including heavy metals and some radioactive debris into the Gulf of Mexico. This allegedly has caused "widespread irreparable damage to the marine and shore environments" including coral reef areas that provide habitats for fish and shellfish.

ITEM: A "government study concludes that more than 200,000 Americans will die before the end of this century because they were exposed to asbestos in earlier years," United Press International reports in December 1981. The wire service notes that "the government has not made public" the report, but it was obtained by journalists.

ITEM: "Most people that die by fire today die because of toxic materials and exposure to breathing the toxics as a result of the fire, not from the flames themselves. 95% or higher die from inhalation of toxic fumes," says Ronald Buckingham, Suffolk County, New York director of fire safety in a television interview in March 1982. Whether it's the Stauffer's Inn tragedy or most other fatal fires, toxic gases given off from "virtually all the furnishings made today" do the killing, he says. The "technology is available to build products that are inherently fire safe," he continues, but this is more expensive and manufacturers prefer cheapness "in order to sell things. Safety in these areas must be federally mandated."

ITEM: DDT was finally banned in the U.S. in 1972 and the birds threatened with extinction by the poison—including the national bird, the bald eagle—are making a comeback. No longer are bird eggs paper-thin as an effect of DDT, in America. Overseas that is not the situation. In Zambia, fish eagle eggs are reported thin "because of DDT in the birds' diet of fish," reports *The New York Times* in October 1981. Fear for the fate of the majestic fish eagle is being voiced. And the head of the Zambian Wildlife Conservation Society, who says DDT being exported into Africa is "being used in an uncontrolled way," notes it is also showing up in dairy products, beef, corn and human milk.

ITEM: "Industrial chemicals have been found in the underground drinking supply of 29% of the cities of over 10,000 people checked in a nationwide survey, the Environmental Protection Agency said yesterday," reports the *Washington Post* in July 1982. It adds: "However, Victor Kimm, head of EPA's drinking water program, said the agency did not regard the report as a big concern."

ITEM: "More than 130 demonstrators, including the Rev. Joseph E. Lowery, president of the Southern Christian Leadership Conference, were arrested today after they tried to block trucks from entering and leaving a PCB dump site in Warren County," reports the Associated Press on September 20, 1982. The State of North Carolina's "decision to dump the toxic wastes . . . has set off a continuing struggle," A.P. notes. Governor James B. Hunt, Jr. defends the dumping and protestors chant "Dump Hunt in the Dump."

It is June 1982, still a silent spring, and President Ronald Reagan declares it "National Pest Control Month."

THE WHITE HOUSE

WASHINGTON

NATIONAL PEST CONTROL MONTH
June, 1982

Mankind has been waging a tug-of-war with pests
since the beginnings of civilization. Sometimes
we win, and sometimes they do -- at least tempo-
rarily. From the vermin-spread Plague of the
Dark Ages to the termite and cockroach problems
of today, pests have been a scourge.

Even in our bountiful land, we cannot afford to
tolerate the disease and destruction they spread.

National Pest Control Month is an excellent time
to focus attention on the persistence of pests
and to discuss how we can all work to contain
and control them.

The National Pest Control Association and the
industry it represents are to be commended
for their participation in this educational
observance.

I encourage everyone to support effective pest
management whenever and wherever possible.

Ronald Reagan

What can be done?
"The epidemic of chemical violence spilling across the land
and waters of America provokes a new patriotism: to stop the

poisoning of the country," declared Ralph Nader, Ronald Bronstein and John Richard in *Who's Poisoning America, Corporate Polluters and their Victims in the Chemical Age.* "It invites a new kind of neighborhood unity: to defend the community, the children and those yet unborn. It highlights the severe deficiencies in our laws, in the flow of information and in the response of our public officials. It reflects a destruction of civilized standards by corporate executives."

"Politics of Poison," a 1979 broadcast on KRON-TV in San Francisco, about dioxin-laden 2,4,5-T, the basic ingredient of Agent Orange and then and now sold in consumer products such as Silvex, Weed-B-Gone and others, began with this introduction: "What if you and your children were receiving tiny doses of a terrible poison—a synthetic chemical so powerful that an ounce could wipe out a million people? Is that too incredible, too bizarre to believe? And if that were happening, wouldn't the government do something about it?"

The *Silent Spring* of Rachel Carson, indeed the issues in the classic 1933 book, *100,000,000 Guinea Pigs, Dangers in Everyday Foods, Drugs, and Cosmetics,* remain with us— with ever greater intensity—to this day and stand to become still more serious in the future because there is *no protection.*

The government is doing virtually nothing about it!

The almighty dollar is the bottom line, and with anything and everything being done in America to make a buck, it doesn't matter who is injured, who is killed. Technology is runaway, uncontrolled, saturating the environment with poisons.

"There is no such thing as a responsible corporate investment," says Lorna Salzman of Friends of the Earth. It's a contradiction in terms. Anything that stands in the way of profit, whether environmental laws or the peoples' health, is trampled on. It's a dog-eat-dog mentality. We're not going to see socially responsible behavior in America until there's a revolution—of people demanding: 'the poisoning will stop.'"

She is for an amendment to the Bill of Rights declaring that every citizen is entitled to "an environment free of harmful substances. That's a basic human right."

She is against *any* government countenance of toxics. "To let the government set standards for known toxics, to sanction the number of illnesses and death, is not moral. No one is entitled to do that."

She insists that the "burden of proof must be on the manufacturers, users and disposers" of materials potentially harmful to show that they are safe "to humans, other life and future generations."

And "any discharge of any toxics," declares Mrs. Salzman, should be met with "absolute and automatic criminal penalties."

Further, she says citizens should be "given the legal power to institute citizens suits without having to prove personal damage," to have the standing as citizens to go into court at all times to sue those who contaminate them and the environment.

The poisons that we have been subjected to are all replaceable by safe materials and processes. Ecologist Barry Commoner speaks of the synthetic "actors" injected by technology into the natural cycle, breaking the delicate "circle of life" and causing effects damaging to life.

"We have broken out of the circle of life, converting its endless cycles into man-made, linear events," Commoner notes. "Man-made breaks into the ecosphere's cycles spew out toxic chemicals, sewage, heaps of rubbish—the testimony to our power to tear the ecological fabric that has, for millions of years, sustained the planet's life . . . If we are to survive, we must understand why this collapse now threatens."

All the toxins—from PCB's to chemical pesticides, herbicides and fertilizers—can be substituted with substances and procedures which harmonize with nature. The only loss in this change would be in the profits of the corporate peddlers of poisons.

This is not a relative matter, not a mosaic of greys, not something involving "cost-benefit."

We are talking of poison. We are talking of resulting mass injuries, cancer and death. We are talking of survival.

The issues are clear and life hinges on the outcome. *The poisoning must end. The Poison Conspiracy must be broken.*

This is a deeply entrenched network and it will not be easy. But there is no choice if we and our descendants are to survive.

Index